Practical Cutaneous Cryosurgery

Practical Cutaneous Cryosurgery

Douglas Torre, M. D.
  Clinical Professor of Medicine (Dermatology)
  Cornell University Medical College
  New York, New York

Ronald R. Lubritz, M.D.
  Clinical Professor of Medicine (Dermatology)
  Tulane University School of Medicine
  New Orleans, Louisiana

Emanuel G. Kuflik, M.D.
  Clinical Associate Professor of Medicine (Dermatology)
  University of Medicine and Dentistry of New Jersey
  New Jersey Medical School, Newark, New Jersey

with a Foreword by
Andrew A. Gage, M.D.
Professor of Surgery
Buffalo School of Medicine
State University of New York
Buffalo, New York

APPLETON & LANGE
Norwalk, Connecticut/San Mateo, California

0-8385-7870-5

Notice: Our knowledge in clinical sciences is constantly changing. As new information becomes available, changes in treatment and in the use of drugs become necessary. The author(s) and the publisher of this volume have taken care to make certain that the doses of drugs and schedules of treatment are correct and compatible with the standards generally accepted at the time of publication. The reader is advised to consult carefully the instruction and information material included in the package insert of each drug or therapeutic agent before administration. This advice is especially important when using new or infrequently used drugs.

Copyright © 1988 by Appleton & Lange
A Publishing Division of Prentice Hall

All rights reserved. This book, or any parts thereof, may not be used or reproduced in any manner without written permission. For information, address Appleton & Lange, 25 Van Zant Street, East Norwalk, Connecticut 06855.

88 89 90 91 92 / 10 9 8 7 6 5 4 3 2 1

Prentice-Hall International (UK) Limited, *London*
Prentice-Hall of Australia Pty. Limited, *Sydney*
Prentice-Hall Canada, Inc., *Toronto*
Prentice-Hall Hispanoamericana, S. A., *Mexico*
Prentice-Hall of India Private Limited, *New Delhi*
Prentice-Hall of Japan, Inc., *Tokyo*
Simon & Schuster Asia Pte. Ltd., *Singapore*
Editora Prentice-Hall do Brasil Ltda., *Rio de Janeiro*
Prentice-Hall, *Englewood Cliffs, New Jersey*

Library of Congress Cataloging-in-Publication Data

Torre, Douglas, 1919-
  Practical cutaneous cryosurgery/Douglas Torre, Ronald R.
Lubritz, Emanuel G. Kuflik; with a foreword by Andrew A. Gage.
    p.   cm.
  Includes bibliographies and index.
  ISBN 0-8385-7870-5
  1. Skin–Surgery.   2. Cryosurgery.   I. Lubritz, Ronald R., 1934-
II. Kuflik, Emanuel G.   III. Title.
  [DNLM: 1. Cryosurgery–methods.   2. Skin–surgery.   3. Skin
Neoplasms–surgery. WR 650 T689p]
RD520.T67 1988
617'.477059–dc19
DNLM/DLC   88-16787
for Library of Congress   CIP

Production Editors: Julie Blum, Mary Beth Miller
Designer: Kathleen Peters Ceconi

PRINTED IN THE UNITED STATES OF AMERICA

*This book is dedicated to our wives
Cathy, Deborah, and Rhoda*

CONTENTS

FOREWORD

Though cryosurgery has long been used in the treatment of skin disease, its importance in medical practice burgeoned only after modern cryosurgical apparatus was developed in 1963 by Dr. Irving Cooper in New York City. In the next few years, wide interest in the application of cryosurgery to various diseases led to the development of diverse types of instrumentation, including devices well suited to the treatment of skin disease. The new techniques of cryosurgery quickly created a need for learning the correct use of the new apparatus.

The authors of this book have contributed substantially to the development of cryosurgery for skin disease. Dr. Douglas Torre is a pioneer in modern cryosurgery. His innovative ideas have found expression in the development of new equipment in the mid 1960s and his techniques have proven useful in dermatologic practice. Dr. Ronald Lubritz has contributed to the development of new cryosurgical techniques and to the teaching of their effective use. The postgraduate educational courses in cryosurgery of the American Academy of Dermatology were developed in 1979 under codirectors Dr. Torre and Dr. Lubritz. Both have been presidents of the American College of Cryosurgery. Dr. Emanuel Kuflik, a long-term participant in the educational activities of the American Academy of Dermatology and the current secretary of the American College of Cryosurgery, has also made important contributions to the development of cryosurgery, and currently directs the American Academy of Dermatology course.

This book is designed for those who wish to use cyrosurgery for the treatment of skin disease. Its content is based largely on educational material that has matured through presentation at the successive postgraduate courses offered at the annual meeting of the American Academy of Dermatology. After providing a foundation in the cryobiologic basis of cryosurgery, the book describes the diverse techniques which have proven useful in cryosurgical practice. The description of complications and results assure its value to those physicians already experienced in cryosurgery. The book will prove to be of substantial value to those who wish to use cryosurgical techniques in their practice.

Andrew A. Gage, M.D.
Professor of Surgery
Buffalo School of Medicine
State University of New York

ACKNOWLEDGMENTS

We would like to acknowledge the assistance and advice of our fellow cryosurgeons who have worked with us in developing the treatment methods outlined in this text and have taught at the courses and lectures given at the American Academy of Dermatology, American College of Cryosurgery, American Society for Dermatological Surgery, and the International Society for Dermatological Surgery meetings. Particularly helpful were Drs. Gloria Graham, Gilberto Castro-Ron, Andrew Gage, Setrag Zacarian, Jack Waller, Richard Elton, Rachel Spiller, and William Spiller.

FIGURE CREDITS

Figures 1-1B and 3-3 reproduced with permission from: Torre DP: Cutaneous cyrosurgery. *J of Cryosurgery* 1968; 1: 202–209.

Figures 1-5B and 2-1 reproduced with permission from: Torre DP: Cyrosurgery, in Andrade R, et al (eds): *Cancer of the Skin: Biology-Diagnosis-Management*. Philadelphia, Saunders, 1976, pp 1569–1587.

Figure 3-6E reproduced with permission from: Torre DP: Instrumentation and monitoring devices in cryosurgery, in Zacarian SA (ed): *Cryosurgery for Skin Cancer and Cutaneous Disorders*. St Louis, Mosby, 1985, pp 31–40.

Figures 3-8A and 3-9 reproduced with permission from: Kuflik EG, Lubritz RR, Torre DP: Cryosurgery. *Dermatologic Clinics* 1984; 2: 319–332.

Figure 3-8B reproduced with permission from: Torre DP: Cryosurgical treatment of epitheliomas using the cone-spray technique. *J Dermatol Surg Oncol* 1977; 3: 433.

Figures 3-10, 6-3A, 6-3B, 6-3C, 6-3D, and 6-7A reproduced with permission from: Torre DP: Cryosurgery of common skin tumors, in Epstein E, Epstein E Jr (eds): *Techniques of Skin Surgery*. Philadelphia, Lea & Febiger, 1979, pp 123–133.

Figures 4-1, 4-2, 4-3, 4-4, 4-5, 7-1A, and 7-1B reproduced with permission from: Torre DP: Cryosurgery of basal cell carcinoma. *J Am Acad Dermatol* 1986; 15: 917–929.

Figures 6-4C and 6-4D courtesy of Dr. Nia Terazakis.

Figures 6-7B and 6-7C reproduced with permission from: Zacarian SA: *Cryosurgical advances in dermatology and tumors of the head and neck*. Springfield, IL, Thomas, 1977, p 65.

Figures 7-3A, 7-3B, 7-3C, 7-5A, 7-5B, and 7-5C reproduced with permission from: Lubritz RR, Torre DP: Cutaneous cryosurgery for nonmalignant and malignant lesions, in Coleman WP, Coleman WP: *Outpatient Surgery of the Skin*. New Hyde Park, NY, Medical Examinations Publishing Co., 1983, pp 188–224.

Figure 7-4C reproduced with permission from Kuflik EG: Cryosurgical treatment of large basal cell carcinomas on the trunk. *J Dermatol Surg Oncol* 1983; 9: 226–230.

Figures 7-6A, 7-6B, 7-6C, and 7-6D reproduced with permission from: Kuflik EG: Cryosurgery for skin cancer. *J Med Soc NJ* 1981; 78: 277–280.

Figures 7-7A, 7-7B, 7-7C, and 7-7D reproduced with permission from: Kuflik EG: CRYO Corner: "Debulking large tumors." *J Dermatol Surg Oncol* 1982; 8: 431–433.

Figures 7-12A and 7-12B reproduced with permission from: Kuflik EG: Cryosurgery for skin cancer. *J Med Soc NJ* 1981; 78: 277–280.

Figures 7-13A and 7-13B reproduced with permission from: Kuflik EG: Cryosurgery for Lentigo Maligna: A report of four cases. *J Dermatol Surg Oncol* 1980; 6: 432–435.

CHAPTER 1

Introduction to Cutaneous Cryosurgery

HISTORY

Cutaneous cryosurgery has an extensive history. Dr. A. Campbell White was the first dermatologist to use cryosurgery, as we now define it, for the treatment of patients. Before the turn of the century, he applied liquid air to skin lesions. He devised and mainly used the *swab* technique in which cotton–wool was wrapped around the end of a stick, then dipped in liquid air, withdrawn, and applied to the lesion (Fig. 1-1A). He also experimented with a *wash bottle spray device* to apply droplets of liquid air onto the skin surface (Fig. 1-1B). Dr. White treated a diversity of lesions including warts, nevi, skin cancers, skin tuberculosis, and even poison ivy dermatitis. The swab technique was later adapted for use with liquid oxygen in the 1920s and with liquid nitrogen in the 1940s. Swab application with liquid nitrogen is still being used today.

Carbon dioxide was first used as a cryogen by Juliusberg, but W. A. Pusey popularized it in the United States during the first decade of the twentieth century. It has been used continuously since then, mainly in the form of "pencils" of solid carbon dioxide carved from blocks or formed by packing crystals into hollow tubes. These crystals are formed when liquid carbon dioxide is released into chamois bags or special containers. Because this cryogen is not as cold as liquid nitrogen, it is not suitable to treat skin cancers and is mainly used for treating warts, keratoses, and angiomas. By combining solid carbon dioxide crystals with ether or acetone a *slush* can be formed and used for surface application to broad areas of the skin. This has been used mainly for treating acne vulgaris and its sequelae.

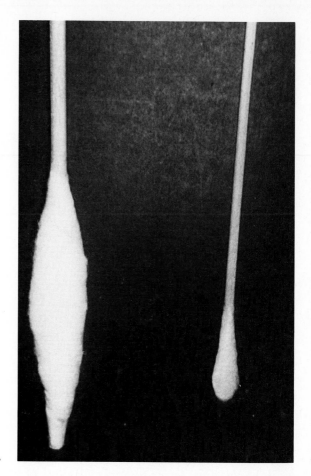

Figure 1-1A. Cotton-tipped swabs for cryogen application.

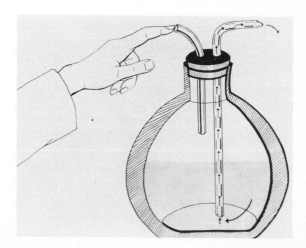

Figure 1-1B. Wash bottle technique for spraying liquid cryogen. In the 1890s Dr. White used liquid air.

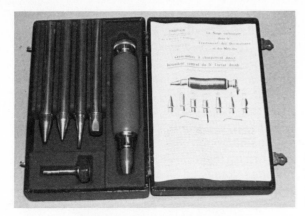

Figure 1-2. Lorent Jacob (French) cryoprobe apparatus (1920s) that used carbon dioxide slush as cryogen.

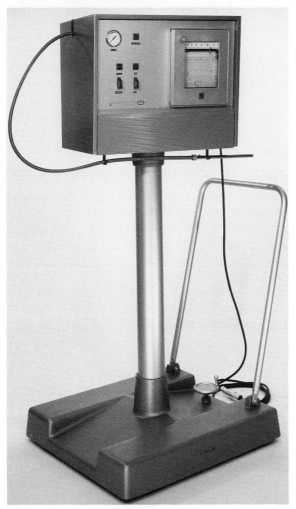

Figure 1-3. Cooper liquid nitrogen cryoprobe (1961) developed by Union Carbide (Linde Division).

The French adapted a carbon dioxide and solvent mixture for *cryoprobe* use, chilling the inside of variously shaped applicators, which then could be applied to skin lesions with controlled pressure due to incorporated spring devices (Fig. 1-2). This cryoprobe method was not fully exploited until the neurosurgeon, Irving Cooper, devised his revolutionary system using liquid nitrogen in the early 1960s (Fig. 1-3).

A simplified cryoprobe for treating skin lesions was reported by Setrag Zacarian in 1965. This consisted of copper cylinders of different sizes that were dipped into liquid nitrogen and then applied to the skin (Fig. 1-4A).

The spray technique, using liquid nitrogen, was devised by Dr. Torre in 1965 (Fig. 1-4B). The early apparatus consisted of an insulated handle attached by a flexible silicone rubber tubing to a 25-liter liquid nitrogen storage tank. Various sized spray tips and cryoprobes could be affixed to the handle (Fig. 1-4C). Later, much smaller, portable hand-held units were devised by Dr. Torre and others (Fig. 1-5). At present, several easy-to-use units with vacuum flasks are available. In dermatology the spray mode is by far the most popular but cryoprobes are used for certain situations. Probes cooled with nitrous oxide are also used when liquid nitrogen is not available or when infrequent use makes liquid nitrogen, which cannot be stored indefinitely, impractical.

Clinical criteria were used for all depth determinations in early cryosurgical procedures and are still used for most procedures today. Instrumentation is also used now to monitor freezing of malignant and certain nonmalignant lesions.

In 1961, H. Brodthagen, in Denmark, published the first extensive studies using pyrometer–thermocouple measurements and devised an apparatus for the accurate placement of thermocouple needles under the skin surface. I. S. Cooper also made extensive use of temperature measurements. In France, Patrick LePivert first suggested, in 1977, the use of measurement of electrical flow through tissue to estimate completeness of freezing in depth. He used an AC current-powered ohmmeter to measure *impedance*. Zacarian and Torre designed smaller, battery-operated (DC) units that measure tissue resistance. Acceptance by the Food and Drug Administration has not yet been obtained for this method of measuring depth dose.

CURRENT USE

Today, cryosurgery is widely used in dermatology and has been established as the treatment method of choice for many cutaneous lesions and as an alternate method in many other situations. It supplements the use of excision, curettage, electrosurgery, chemosurgery, laser surgery, and ionizing irradiation, and it can often be used in combination with these methods. Its applicability, as well as its many advantages and few disadvantages, are discussed in those chapters dealing with specific skin lesions (Table 1-1).

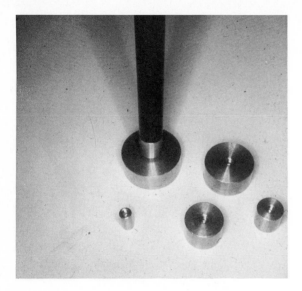

Figure 1-4A. Zacarian copper discs (1964).

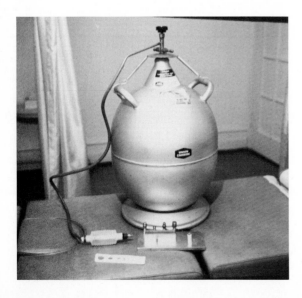

Figure 1-4B. Torre prototype of cryoprobe spray unit for liquid nitrogen (1965) developed by Union Carbide.

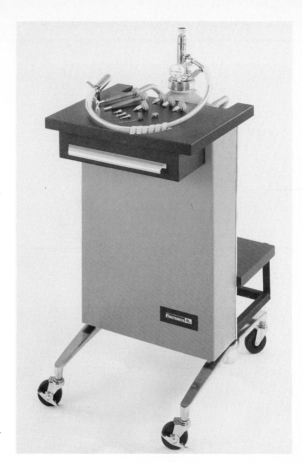

Figure 1-4C. CE-8 unit developed by Union Carbide and Frigitronics based on Torre prototype (1969).

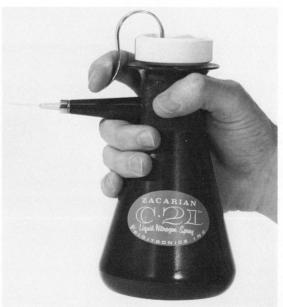

Figure 1-5A. Zacarian C-21 hand-held spray unit developed by Frigitronics, Inc. (1969).

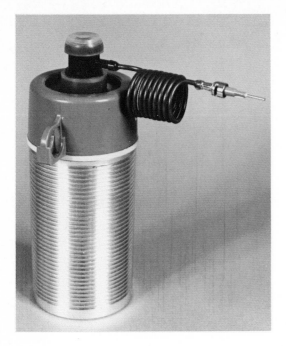

Figure 1-5B. Lubritz-Johns "Foster Froster" (1975).

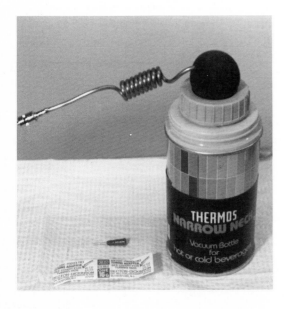

Figure 1-5C. Torre "do-it-yourself" hand-held apparatus designed for the American Academy of Dermatology Cryosurgery home study course (1970s).

TABLE 1-1. LESIONS BEING TREATED BY CRYOSURGERY

Cryosurgery Treatment of Choice

Basal cell carcinoma (superficial multicentric type)	Periungual warts
Dermatofibroma	Porokeratosis (actinic)
Keratosis (actinic)	Porokeratosis (plantar)
Lentigo (actinic—benign)	Sebaceous hyperplasia
Leukoplakia	Verruca (digitate)
Mucocoele	

Cryosurgery as an Alternate Method of Treatment (sometimes combined with other methods)

Acne pits	Kaposi's sarcoma
Acne pustules and cysts	Keloid
Acrochordon	Keratoacanthoma
Adenoma sebaceum (pringle)	Keratosis (arsenical)
Angiofibroma	Keratosis (seborrheic)
Angiokeratoma	Leiomyoma
Angiomas	Leishmaniasis
Basal cell carcinoma (nodular)	Lentigo maligna
Papular	Lupus erythematosus
ulcerative	Lupus vulgaris
cystic	Molluscum contagiosum
Bowen's disease	Myxoid cysts
Carbuncle	Neurofibroma
Chloasma	Nevus
Chrondrodermatitis	Porokeratosis (mibelli)
Clear cell acanthosis	Prurigo nodularis
Condylomata accuminata	Pyogenic granuloma
Cylindroma	Rhinophyma
Eccrine poroma	Sarcoid
Elastosis perforans serpiginosa	Squamous cell carcinoma
Eosinphilic granuloma	Steatocystoma multiplex
Granuloma annulare	Syringoma
Granuloma faciale	Trichoepithelioma
Granuloma (mycobacterial)	Verruca planae
Hidradenoma	Verruca plantaris
Hidradenitis	Verruca vulgaris
Histiocytoma	Xanthelasma

SELECTED READING

Allington HV: Liquid nitrogen in the treatment of skin diseases. Calif Med 72:153, 1950

Brodthagen H: Local freezing of the skin by carbon dioxide snow. Munksgaurd, Copenhagen, 1961

Cooper IS, Lee AS: Cryostatic congelation: A system for producting a limited controlled region of cooling or freezing of biologic tissues. J Nerv Ment Dis 133:259, 1961

Irvine HG, Turnacliff DD: Liquid oxygen in dermatology. Arch Dermat Syph 19:270, 1929

Torre D: Alternate cryogens for cryosurgery. J Dermatol Surg Oncol 1:56, 1975

Torre D: New York: Cradle of cryosurgery. NY State J Med 67:465, 1967

White AC: Possibilities of liquid air to the physician. JAMA 36:426, 1901

White AC: Liquid air in medicine and surgery. Med Rec 56:109, 1899

Whitehouse HH: Liquid air in dermatology: Its indications and limitations. JAMA 49(5):371, 1907

CHAPTER *2*

Cryobiology

When discussing cryobiology it should be remembered that there are degrees of difference when treating malignant or nonmalignant lesions with cryosurgery. Clinical treatment methods in large part depend on and have been derived from understanding and using these differences. Treatment of malignant lesions depend on the destructive effects of cryosurgery; successful treatment of nonmalignant conditions, in most instances, depends on minimizing these same factors.

When treating benign epidermal lesions the excellent results obtained depend on the fact that a mild amount of freezing causes separation of the epidermis from the dermis above the PAS-positive membrane, thus allowing for ablation of the lesion and rapid reepithelization of the wound with healthy cells lining the epidermal appendages and surrounding epithelium (Fig. 2-1).

When treating deep tumors or malignancies, good results from cryosurgery come from the fact that cellular components are more susceptible to cold injury than are stromal components.

PHYSICS OF CRYOBIOLOGY

In discussing the elementary physics of cryobiology it is important to remember that the flow of temperature is always from the warmer to the colder object. Cold is, therefore, a negative factor. Placing a cold applicator on a

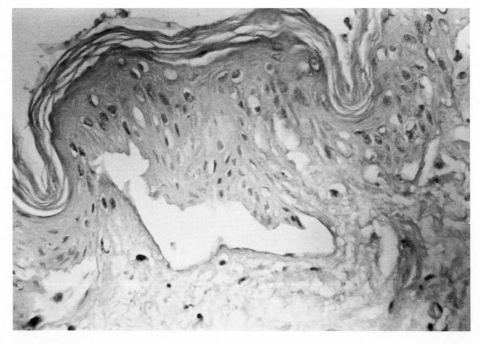

Figure 2-1. Photomicrograph of separation of the epidermis from the dermis above the PAS-positive membrane after mild cryosurgery.

warm target produces a temperature difference. The cold applicator is described as a heat sink. When applied to the warmer skin, it withdraws heat from the tissue. The capacity of a heat sink varies with its size, its composition, and the temperature difference. Conductivity factors are also important. Air is a poor conductor, water is a fair conductor, and metal is a good conductor. Ice is a better conductor than water. When an iceball is created, the process goes faster after the ice forms. Thermal gradients are also set up within the iceball, and both of these factors are considered when treatment methods are used.

The junction between the heat sink and the target is the *interface*. This junction is important in cryosurgical procedures because interface factors play an important role not only with our treatment techniques, but also in the results produced. Remembering that the conductivity factors can predict, for instance, that if a solid probe is placed on an uneven dry surface, poor contact results. But if a liquid or spray is used as the cryogen source, one gets a good contact on the target surface. If a pointed probe is pressed into the skin, this increases the interface surface and thus increases heat transfer.

DESTRUCTIVE EFFECTS OF FREEZING

The effect of cold on human tissue depends on several factors: the rate of temperature fall, the rate of rewarming, the solute concentration, the length of time the cells are exposed to a below-freezing temperature, and the coldest temperature reached in the target tissue. It has been shown that slow cooling produces extracellular ice. This is not as damaging as rapid cooling, which produces intracellular ice. Rapid cooling of the target tissue is, therefore, desirable. The rate of rewarming or thaw, however, should proceed slowly. Chemicals within the tissue concentrate as ice forms and this chemical insult adds to the destructive effects of crystal formation. With a slow thaw, there is an increased concentration of electrolytes over a longer time and recrystallization or grain growth is also produced. This is more damaging to the cells. With repeated freeze–thaw cycles, maximum destructive effects are produced.

For many years dermatologic cryosurgeons used −25C to −30C as a target for the coldest temperature reached at the base of a basal cell carcinoma. New evidence in recent years, however, has shown that this temperature is not adequate, except for superficial lesions. Present day techniques require that the temperature reach at least −50C when treating deeper basal cell carcinomas and all malignancies with a potential for metastasis. This is the temperature at which skin is completely frozen. Freezing to a temperature of below −60C does not increase destruction. Of the more commonly available cryogens, only liquid nitrogen is adequate to reach the temperature for maximum destructive effects. Other cryogens can and have been used to

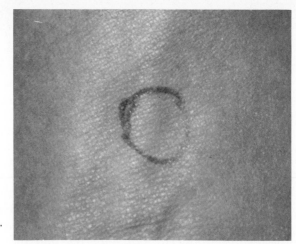

Figure 2-2. Mild application of cold to skin (normal wrist). **A.** Target margin marked.

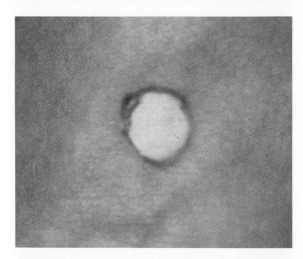

Figure 2-2B. Target area frozen.

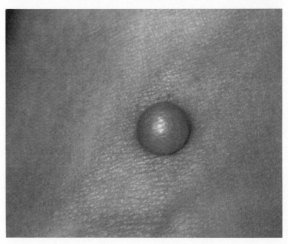

Figure 2-2C. Postoperative bullous reaction.

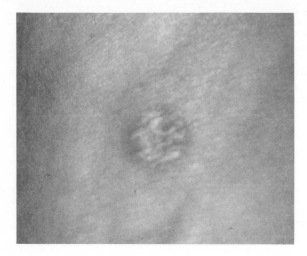

Figure 2-2D. Early healing phase with depigmentation.

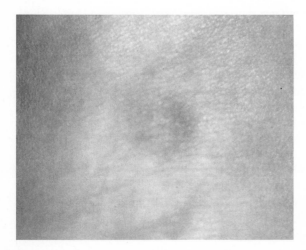

Figure 2-2E. Late healing phase with temporary hyperpigmentation.

TABLE 2-1. TEMPERATURES OF CRYOGENS

| | Temperature (C) | |
Cryogen	Boiling point when used in closed cryoprobe system	Applied to skin in open atmosphere
Liquid nitrogen	−196	−196
Nitrous oxide	−88.4	—
Carbon dioxide	—	−78.5
Halocarbon 22	−40.8	−70*
Halocarbon 12	−29.8	−60*
Halocarbon 114	—	−30*

*Approximate temperatures.

treat nonmalignancies, but they are not adequate for the treatment of malignant lesions (Table 2-1).

In clinical application, any cryosurgical method should:

1. Produce rapid cooling of the target tissue.
2. Extend the iceball beyond the target margins for sufficient cooling of the entire target.
3. Allow for slow thawing.
4. Allow for repeat freeze–thaw cycles, if necessary.

CLINICAL EFFECTS

The clinical effects of cryosurgery should be familiar to the clinician (Figs. 2-2 and 2-3). This knowledge serves not only to assure that the cryosurgical procedure proceeded correctly, but it also is necessary to explain to patients what to expect. At first erythema and urtication occur. This is caused by histamine release and usually begins within a few minutes after starting the procedure. Edema then follows because of blood vessel damage. This takes place within a few minutes and peaks at 12 to 36 hours. Vesiculation develops after urtication and can be either serous or hemorrhagic; exudation and sloughing of tissue is a part of this reaction. Crusting occurs after a few days, and depending on the depth of freeze, it can last 1 to 4 weeks, or even longer. Cellular regrowth usually starts within 48 hours.

Cryosurgery produces a selective destruction of tissue. Cellular elements are more susceptible than are stromal elements. This allows for destruction of tumors overlying and invading bone and cartilage. It also allows for freezing of large blood vessels without their rupture, and accounts for nerve regeneration after injury from cold. On occasion, however, it can also account for superficial nerve damage. Melanocytes are more susceptible than keratinocytes, and their destruction can lead to depigmentation. Repigmentation occurs from the migration of melanocytes from the margins or from undamaged melanocytes in hair follicles.

DELIVERY OF THE CRYOGEN

There are two basic methods of delivering the cryogen, usually liquid nitrogen, to the target lesion: cryospray and cryoprobe techniques. Modification of these methods, such as the cone-spray technique, are discussed in Chapter 3.

When using the cryospray technique the cryogen is applied through an open spray tip that is held directly over the target site. The spray is always confined within the borders of the lesion, and various spray patterns can be used.

A flat cryoprobe applied with pressure results in a deeper depth of freeze in comparison to the lateral spread of freeze obtained with the cryospray method. The probe surface is cooled either by previous immersion in the cryogen or by circulating the cryogen within it. In this way, a heat sink is created, and heat is transferred from the treatment site to the probe. Various-shaped probes can be used and each produces a slightly different shaped iceball (Fig. 2-4). For example, a pointed tip probe produces an iceball that is deeper than its radius on the surface, whereas a rounded probe, pushed firmly against the skin, produces an iceball approximating a hemisphere. A small, flat probe (5 to 25 mm), applied with mild pressure, produces an iceball that has a lateral spread of freeze approximately equal to the central depth of freeze. To estimate the iceball shape and size when treating skin lesions the formula $DF = LSF$ (depth of freeze equals lateral spread of freeze) is used. This is explained in greater detail in Chapter 4.

It is advisable to determine the iceball patterns developed by each probe or cone. This is most easily done with agar or potato models. The probe is placed on the surface of the model and freezing is carried out until the lateral spread of freeze on the surface reaches a certain point, for instance, 5 mm beyond the margin of the cylinder. The procedure is timed and then the model is transected so the cross section of the depth of freeze can be seen (Fig. 2-5). With the potato model, this frozen area will turn brown after 30 to 60 minutes, therefore, pictorial records are easy to keep. It is also possible to place thermocouple needles in the model to register temperatures in relation to freezing pattern. The potato model is not comparable to skin for measuring electrical resistances because the electrolytes are different. To compare lateral spread of freeze and depth of freeze with electrical resistance measurements, a meat model is necessary.

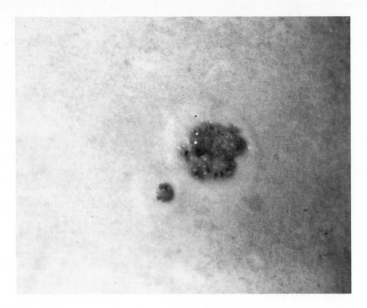

Figure 2-3. Severe application of cold (basal cell carcinoma). **A.** Urtication 10 minutes postfreeze.

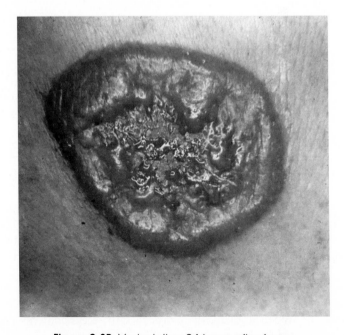

Figure 2-3B. Vesiculation 24 hours after freeze.

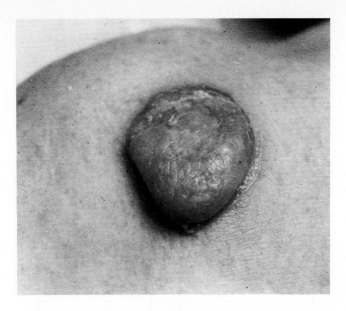

Figure 2-3C. Gelatinous reaction 48 hours after freeze.

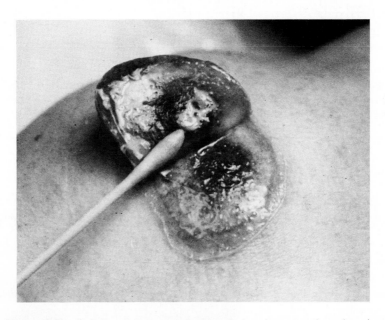

Figure 2-3D. Gelatinous mass peeled back showing granulomatous base.

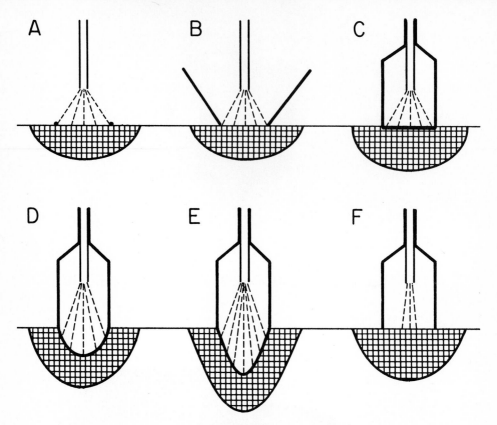

Figure 2-4. Application modes with corresponding iceball shape. **A.** Open spray. **B.** Cone spray. **C.** Flat cryoprobe. **D.** Rounded cryoprobe. **E.** Pointed cryoprobe. **F.** Open-end cryoprobe.

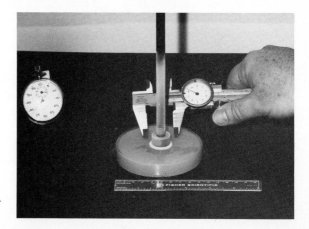

Figure 2-5. Learning iceball dimensions. **A.** Cryoprobe applied to agar plate.

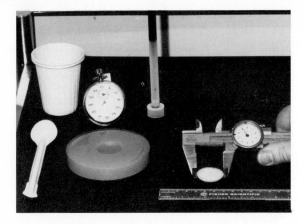

Figure 2-5B. Hemispheric ice-ball removed from plate for measurements of width and depth.

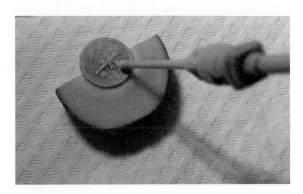

Figure 2-5C. Potato model with dime used to simulate probe effect.

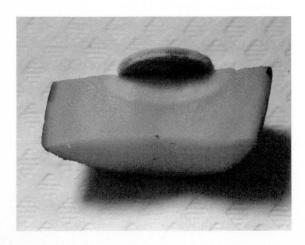

Figure 2-5D. Lateral spread of freeze and depth of freeze easily discernable.

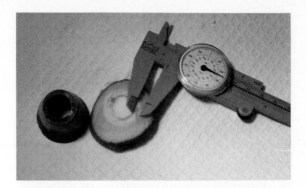

Figure 2-5E. Lateral spread of freeze being measured.

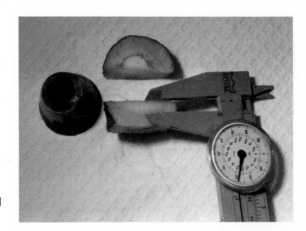

Figure 2-5F. Depth of iceball being measured.

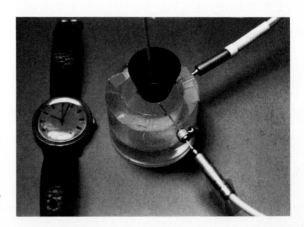

Figure 2-5G. Use of known depth thermocouple to determine isotherms within iceball to be formed in agar gel.

SELECTED READING

Meryman HT: Review of biologic freezing. In Cryobiology, Meryman HT (ed). New York, Academic Press, 1966

Gill W, DaCosta J, Fraser J: The control and predictability of a cryolesion. Cryobiology 6:347, 1970

SELECTED READINGS

CHAPTER 3

Equipping an Office for Cryosurgery

An important aspect for cryosurgery is a basic understanding of cryosurgical equipment. A cryosurgical unit actually consists of a dewar tank, the delivery mechanism, and the spray tips or probes (Table 3-1). This chapter briefly describes the different cryogens and apparatus available today. It offers information that may be helpful for the beginner, for the physician wanting a back-up or replacement unit, or for those wishing to obtain additional units.

CRYOGENIC AGENTS

Liquid Nitrogen

Holding Containers
Liquid nitrogen is the cryogen of choice for dermatologic cryosurgery; therefore, when setting up an office the availability of this cryogen should be determined. In most urban areas liquid nitrogen is supplied by welding supply companies as this liquid is used for inert gas shielding in the welding process. The companies deliver the liquid to the medical offices and pour it into the holding containers (dewars) (Fig. 3-1). Because the labor of delivery is part of the expense, infrequent deliveries are optimal. Holding dewars of 25 to 35 liters are most practical for office use. The more expensive the dewar the longer the holding time, size for size. For instance, a Union Carbide 34XT (extended-time refrigerator) has an evaporation rate of only 0.1 liter per day.

TABLE 3-1. BASIC EQUIPMENT FOR ROUTINE OFFICE CRYOSURGERY

Dewar storage tank (25–30 L) withdrawal device or tiltstand

Hand-held cryosurgical unit

Set of neoprene or otoscope cones

Jaeger retractor for eye protection

Plastic eye shields or goggles

Set of cryoprobes (optional)

If malignant lesions are to be treated add
    Second cryosurgical unit for stand-by
    Pyrometer–thermocouple apparatus with at least two thermocouple-tipped hypo-
       dermic needles.

The 34HC (high-capacity refrigerator) has an evaporation rate of 0.17 liters per day, and the cheaper 35LD, 0.32 liters per day. Dewars can be purchased outright or in some instances rented from the company supplying the liquid nitrogen.

In an active practice, a 25-liter supply of liquid nitrogen would be delivered at intervals of 2 to 6 weeks depending on the frequency of use and the quality of the dewars. In rural areas, liquid nitrogen is available from sources that supply it for storage of semen for artificial insemination of cattle and other animals. When delivery of liquid nitrogen is not available, it is sometimes available in small quantities from universities, hospitals, or commercial laboratories. In this instance a supply in 3- to 10-liter dewars with handles for use in the office might be obtained.

Transferring Liquid Nitrogen

Several devices are available to transfer liquid nitrogen from the storage dewar into the cryosurgical unit. Pouring by hand is possible from small storage dewars (10 liters or smaller). Pouring stands are available for larger containers (Fig. 3-2). For the units larger than 10 liters, however, some transfer device is indicated. The simplest is a dipper, but most dermatologists prefer a spigot-type device. Most of these units use the gas pressure developed by the boil-off of the liquid in the dewar to pressurize the transfer, therefore, there is a time lag between the insertion of the withdrawal device (after the storage tank is filled) and sufficient pressure is built-up to transfer the liquid. This pressure seal must be broken if unused nitrogen is to be poured back into the storage dewar at the end of a treatment session.

Solidified Carbon Dioxide

If liquid nitrogen is not available, limited cryosurgery can be accomplished with solid carbon dioxide obtained at the time of use from ice cream purveyors, from pencils made from stored gas cylinders (Joule-Thompson effect), or from Kidde apparatus with miniature cylinders (Fig. 3-3.)

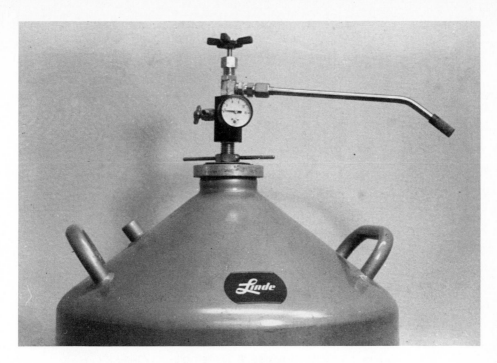

Figure 3-1. Storage dewar for liquid nitrogen with dispenser top (Linde).

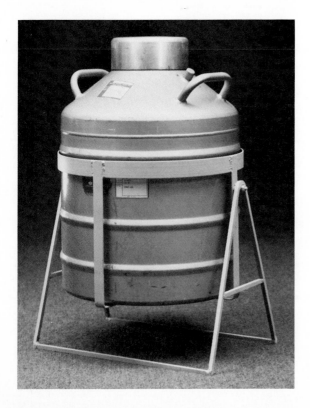

Figure 3-2. Storage dewar on rocker base.

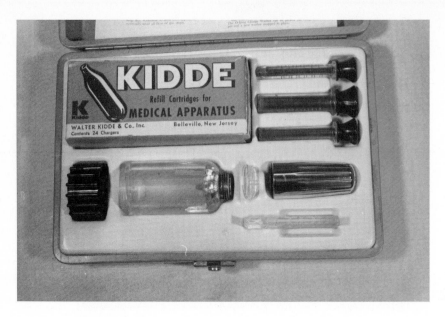

Figure 3-3. Carbon dioxide. **A.** Kidde carbon dioxide kit.

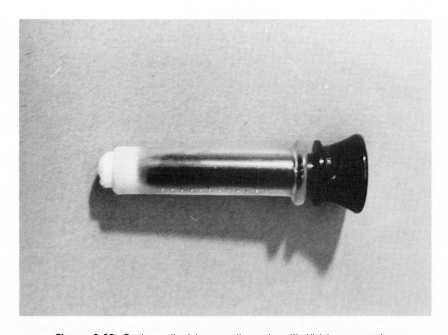

Figure 3-3B. Carbon dioxide pencil made with Kidde apparatus.

Nitrous Oxide

Nitrous oxide apparatus is also available. This cryogen can be stored indefinitely and is usually used in cryoprobe mode (Fig. 3-4). One available apparatus furnishes a spray mode option; however, due to the law of partial pressure of gases, when nitrous oxide liquid is sprayed onto a surface in an open air environment, the droplets do not vaporize but become solid particles and build-up on the surface or fly in all directions. Only by surrounding the droplets with nitrous oxide gas, using a cup-shaped device, will the droplets vaporize on the skin surface. As the minimum temperature reached is about $-80C$, this apparatus is not recommended for treating malignant lesions. Thus, liquid nitrogen is still the only cryogen recommended for the treatment of malignancies.

Fluorocarbon Sprays

Several fluorocarbon sprays are available but two have been found most useful for dermatologic use. Fluorocarbon 114 is marketed as "Frigiderm" by Brachvogel and produces a temperature in the $-30C$ to $-35C$ range when sprayed on the skin surface. Fluorocarbon 12 in a siphon can with nozzle extension is sold for dermatopathologic use as "Cryokwik" (Damon-IEC Division) and produces a skin surface temperature of $-60C$ (Fig. 3-5).

Fluorocarbon sprays can be used for:

1. Calibrating thermocouples (Fluorocarbon 12 at $-60C$).
2. Topical analgesia for minor surgical procedures such as incision and drainage of pustules (Fluorocarbon 114 at $-30C$ to $-35C$).
3. Firming skin surface for dermabrasion (Fluorocarbon 114).
4. Treating acne pustules and cysts (Fluorocarbon 114).
5. Exfoliating skin surfaces for acne pitting, without dermabrasion (Fluorocarbon 12).
6. Treating large plaques of psoriasis, particularly of the scalp (Fluorocarbon 12).
7. Cryosurgical treatment of superficial epidermal lesions such as actinic keratoses and seborrheic keratoses (Fluorocarbon 12).

Caution is advised with these products, as it is possible to produce scarring and permanent depigmentation. In our experience, postinflammatory hyperpigmentation surrounding the treated area is greater with fluorocarbon sprays than with the use of liquid nitrogen. Fluorocarbon vapors should be vented away from operators as well as the patient as cardiac toxicity from chronic inhalation has been reported.

CRYOSURGICAL EQUIPMENT

Cryosurgical apparatus has improved substantially over the last 15 years from a safety standpoint and performance. The delivery mechanism, or de-

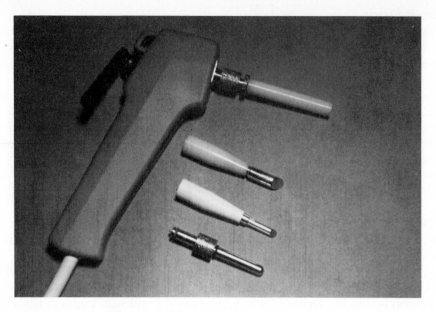

Figure 3-4. Nitrous oxide cryosurgical unit.

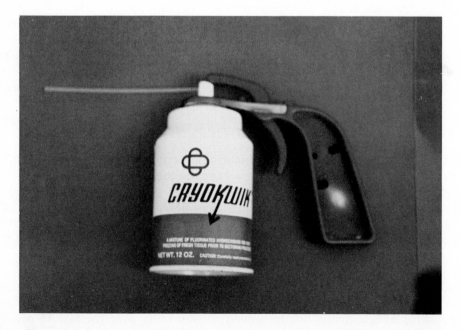

Figure 3-5. Fluorocarbon 12 siphon dispenser can (Cryokwik) (Damon-IEC Division).

vice, is attached to the filled dewar whether it be a hand-held, a table top, or a floor model unit.

When shopping for cryosurgical equipment one should select a unit that is well-constructed, safe, easy to handle, has the desired holding capacity, and adaptable for use with a variety of accessories. It is advisable to have more than one unit in case of malfunction or *ice-up* of the primary unit. The pattern differences of the spray can be tested by spraying on a blotter held in a vertical position and checking for splatter or drip. Spraying should be continued for several minutes to check how fast the instrument *ices up* or starts spraying large drops of liquid.

Surprisingly, the cost of the latest generation of equipment is very reasonable. A potential buyer should visit the exhibits at various meetings, and get the feel of the different units on display.

Operation of Units

All liquid nitrogen cryosurgical units operate by evaporating liquid nitrogen in the closed dewar, placing the contents under pressure. This pressure is then used to force the liquid nitrogen out in the form of a spray. A safety relief valve exists to prevent overpressurization. To activate, a trigger mechanism is depressed allowing the pressure to force the liquid nitrogen to flow up the delivery tube, through the flow valve, and out the nozzle to the tip.

Cryosurgical Devices

For office use, the choice of liquid nitrogen instruments lies between a hand-held unit, a table-top, portable unit, and a small floor model unit.

Hand-held Units

The hand-held units are by far the most popular (Figs. 3-6A through 3-6F). They are lightweight, contain a small amount of liquid nitrogen, and may need refilling during the course of the day. They hold approximately 0.5 to 1.5 liters, and some are self-pressurizing. The units operate at a constant low pressure for immediate use. Most models are available with optional accessories. Some have the capability of being fitted with interchangeable luer-lok tips.

Table-top Units

The table-top unit manufactured by Frigitronics is the CS-76 (Fig. 3-7A). It is an attractive piece of equipment and excellent for treating malignant tumors. Once the spray stream is established, it continues unabated for a longer time than the hand-held units, and can be used for prolonged, continuous or intermittent treatment. It also allows for regulation of the volume of the nitrogen spray. It has several other characteristics that should be evaluated by the user. The unit is a two-tank system and is more difficult to fill (and to empty back into the storage container if all liquid nitrogen is not

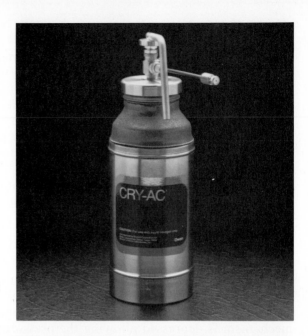

Figure 3-6. Hand-held liquid nitrogen units. **A.** CRY-AC (Brymill).

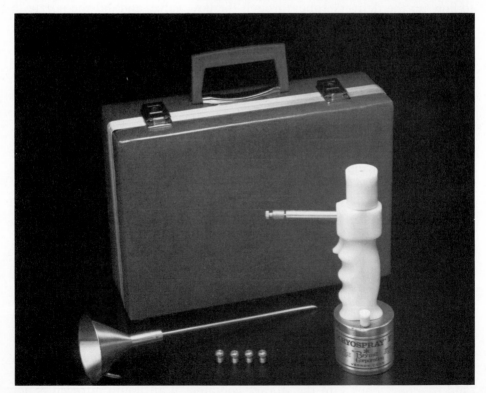

Figure 3-6B. Kryospray II (Brymill).

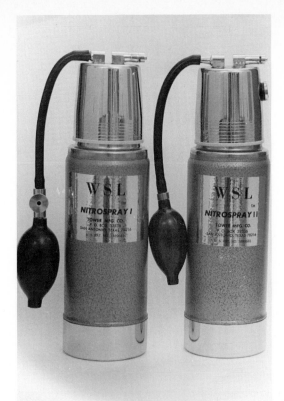

Figure 3-6C. WSL Nitrospray I and II (Tower).

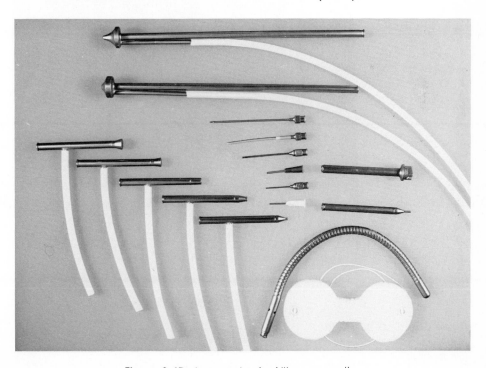

Figure 3-6D. Accessories for Nitrospray units.

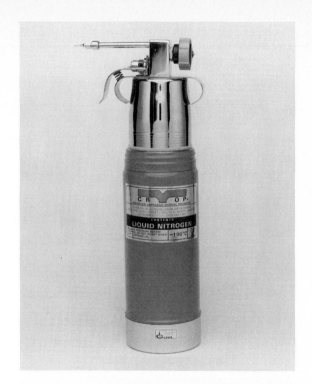

Figure 3-6E. CRYOP (Gilmore).

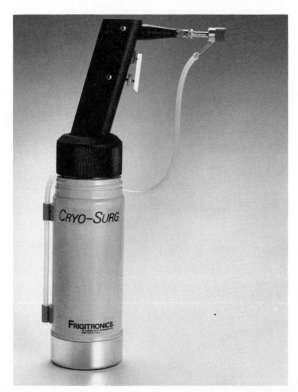

Figure 3-6F. Cryo-Surg, with open-end cryoprobe attached (Frigitronics).

consumed). It uses more nitrogen than the smaller units because one tank is used to pressurize the other. When the trigger is activated there is an almost immediate release of spray from the nozzle, but after a few seconds this spray decreases as the delivery line between the dewar and the nozzle cools down and does not become steady for about 30 to 40 seconds. It is less portable than the hand-held units but is handier when working in areas with limited access, such as the perineal area. One model provides a built-in pyrometer for ease in treatment.

Floor Model Units

The floor model devices hold more liquid nitrogen, between 10 and 30 liters, and maintain a greater pressure than the smaller units. Because they are bulkier, a wheeled base allows for mobility. These units are designed primarily for operating room use.

SPRAY TIPS AND PROBES

All cryosurgical units can be fitted with various spray tips and probes. These are manufactured in a multitude of sizes and shapes for use in specific areas and depending on the size and type of the lesions. Some have interchangeable luer-lok fittings and some do not. One should be advised that when purchasing a back-up or replacement unit, the same accessories should be workable on both units.

Spray Tips

Bypass tips, which allow for a continuous stream of liquid nitrogen to be vented while small amounts are passing through the tiny orifices, should be obtained if a fine spray (20 to 25 gauge bore) is to be used (Fig. 3-7B). Otherwise, dull tip needles or catheter adapters of 15, 16, 17, or 18 gauge bore are satisfactory.

Truncated Cones

Truncated neoprene cones and otoscope cones are quite helpful and inexpensive (Fig. 3-8). The smaller neoprene cones (5, 11, and 18 mm openings) are available from Arthur H. Thomas Co., and are the most useful. Disposable otoscope cones can be used, but we have found that the autoclavable set with 2, 3, 4, 5, and 9 mm openings (Welch-Allen) are superior.

Open-End Probes

Several companies have optional open-end cylinder devices that attach directly to the unit (Fig. 3-6F). These so-called open-end probes vary in size and in the iceball produced on the skin in comparision to the iceball produced by spraying evenly into an open truncated cone placed on the skin. In these devices, the central opening sprays nitrogen onto the skin in the center rather

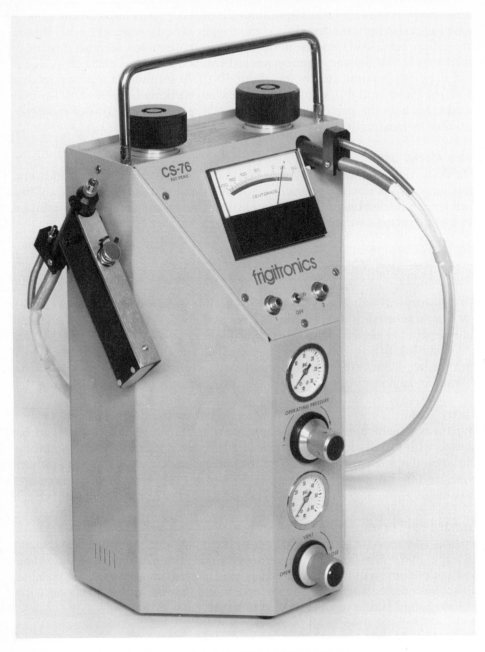

Figure 3-7. Table-top units. **A.** CS-76 (Frigitronics).

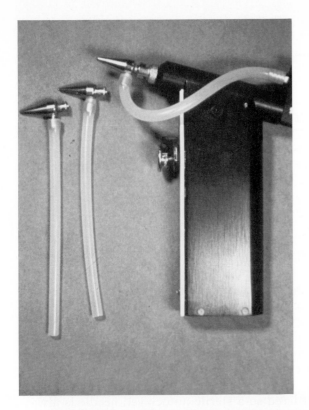

Figure 3-7B. Bypass spray tips (Frigitronics).

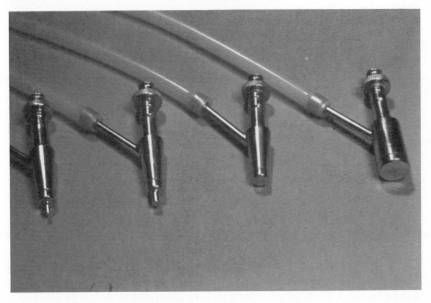

Figure 3-7C. Cryoprobes (Frigitronics).

than near the enclosed periphery of the lesion, changing the dimensions of the iceball when measured by lateral spread beyond the periphery of the cylinder. These devices should be used in conjunction with thermocouple–pyrometer or electrical tissue resistance depth-dose systems.

Cryoprobes

Cryoprobes are available with most cryosurgical units and can be either flat, pointed, or rounded (Fig. 3-7C). The fine-tipped probe is the most useful as it can be used to treat sebaceous hyperplasia, milia, and small flat warts. The flat-end cylindrical probes are used by some physicians to treat tumors. The lateral spread of freeze is easy to measure as it extends peripherally from the probe. Rounded-end probes are useful in treating mucous cysts of the lip, myxoid cysts on the fingers and toes, and vascular lesions.

THERMOCOUPLE–PYROMETER SYSTEM

To treat malignant skin lesions or deep tumors it is necessary to determine the proper depth dose. At the present time, thermocouple–pyrometer systems are standard (Fig. 3-9). Pyrometers with a downside range to −70C are the most accurate as the 0C to −60C range is the one being monitored. An instrument with a device allowing switching to more than one channel is useful when several points are being monitored on one lesion. The 25-gauge thermocouple-tipped needle with a 1-inch length is the most useful size. Several needles should be ordered so a sterile autoclaved needle is always available.

ELECTRICAL TISSUE RESISTANCE

An electrical tissue resistance measuring apparatus is being used experimentally by a number of dermatologists and cryosurgeons but is not yet available commercially. Such a system has some advantages over the thermocouple–pyrometer system and may complement or even replace this system in the future.

PROTECTIVE DEVICES

Protective devices are available to cover vital areas. The eyes, inner canthi, external auditory canal, and nares are critical areas that must be protected during spray freezing from inadvertent spray or liquid nitrogen droplets that could accumulate. Purchasable items include foam or plastic eye goggles, styrofoam, plastic spoons, cotton, or tongue blades. One useful item is the Jaeger retractor, which can be used as an eye shield or to cover the ear canal (Fig. 3-10).

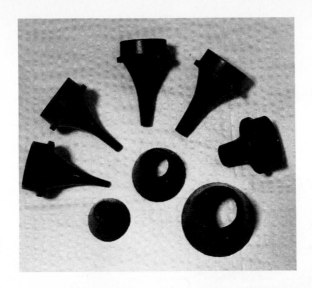

Figure 3-8. Surface limiting devices. **A.** Otoscope and neoprene cones used in restricted spray technique.

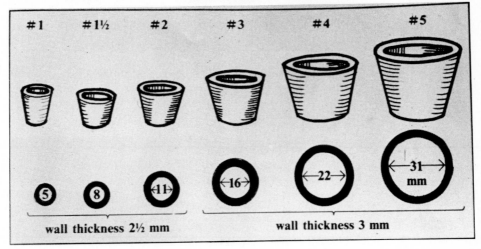

#1 #1½ #2 #3 #4 #5

←5→ ←8→ ←11→ ←16→ ←22→ ←31 mm→

wall thickness 2½ mm   wall thickness 3 mm

Figure 3-8B. Dimensions of fenestrated neoprene cones (Arthur Thomas Co.).

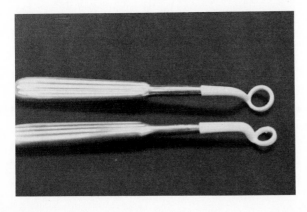

Figure 3-8C. Insulated pressure rings.

39

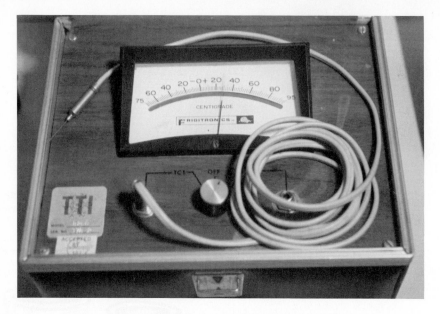

Figure 3-9. Pyrometer-thermocouple apparatus (Frigitronics).

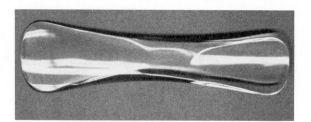

Figure 3-10. Eye protection devices. **A.** Jaeger retractor.

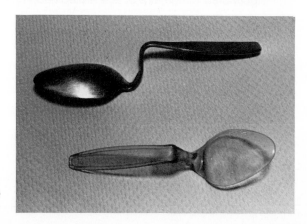

Figure 3-10B. Bent handle spoons.

SELECTED READING

Torre D: Instrumentation and monitoring devices in cryosurgery. In Zacarian SA
(ed): Cryosurgery for Skin Cancer and Cutaneous Disorders. St. Louis, C. V. Mosby,
1985

CHAPTER *4*

Depth Dose Measurement

In treating lesions with cryosurgery it is necessary to estimate within reasonable limits the extent and depth of destruction or alterations that will follow the procedure. Like x-ray or other particle beam modalities, cryosurgery is a *field therapy* and delivers a sublethal or lethal amount of physical insult to tissues within the area treated. The ability to predict these changes at the time of delivery of the insult is of value in treating all lesions, but is critically important in treating malignant tissues. This goal should also be met by the smallest dose that will halt all malignant cells with a minimum alteration on nonmalignant tissue as good functional cosmetic end results are dependent on this.

TARGET TEMPERATURE

The type of dose delivered varies with the target tissue being treated. In treating benign lesions the *dose* can be milder than when treating malignant lesions. For instance, to treat epidermal lesions, such as actinic keratoses, a mild dose that would cause separation of the epidermis from the dermis above the PAS-positive membrane is all that is needed. This dose might be on the order of −15C delivered 1 mm deep for a thin lesion, or 2 to 3 mm deep for a thicker lesion. To treat a malignant lesion with metastatic potential, the dose might involve producing −60C at a depth of 1 cm or more. Cellular damage occurs in the 0C to −60C range, therefore, temperatures lower than −60C do not add to the damage. Repeated freeze-thaw cycles, however, do increase the lethality of the cryosurgical procedures. When treating basal cell carcinomas that do not penetrate through the dermis, experience has shown that it is not necessary to subject the entire tumor to −60C. A milder dose in the −25C to −30C range, delivered to the base of the tumor, produces a satisfactory cure rate with maximum cosmetic end result. Using this dose does not count on total destruction of malignant cells by freezing insult alone. The effect of this amount of cold on the vasculature probably plays a significant role. For practical purposes we limit this milder dose treatment to lesions with a depth of 3 mm or less. Deeper lesions and lesions with metastatic capability should receive the full cell-lethal dose of −50C to −60C to the deepest portion and repeated freeze–thaw cycles.

TARGET AREA

After determining the proper dose, the extent of the area to be targeted must be defined. Unlike excisional surgery, the whole target area is not available for microscopic examination to determine whether the entire tumor has been removed. The extent of the tumor, both peripherally and in depth, must be defined *before* the cryosurgical procedure is carried out. This usually is done by clinical procedures, such as inspection, palpation, and ballottement, and occasional use of curettage. Multiple small biopsies are sometimes taken to determine the extent of a tumor.

TARGET DOSE

Once the extent of the lesion being treated has been estimated, it is necessary to apply the treatment with the proper dose. Judging the proper dose can usually be accomplished by clinical means. If cold is evenly applied to the confines of the surface of the lesion, the spread of freezing on the surface beyond the limits of the lesion becomes apparent. This represents the surface measurement of the three-dimensional ice-ball being formed (Fig. 4-1). The outer margin represents the 0 degree isotherm. The isotherm at various distances from the treated area can be measured by surface thermocouples or can be estimated from known data about the temperature of the cryogen and the rate at which the iceball is formed.

It is also possible to estimate the downward extension of the iceball by measuring its lateral extension (lateral spread of freeze or LSF) (Fig. 4-2). In fact, the depth under the center of the iceball nearly approximates its lateral extension. As with the surface extension of the iceball, the isotherms within the iceball are dependent on the rate of freezing. Thus, we can estimate the lateral and deep effect of the cold that was applied to the surface by measuring the LSF and timing it (freeze time or FT). This clinical dose determination is used for benign lesions and for basal cell carcinomas less than 3 mm in depth (Fig. 4-3).

When treating malignant lesions deeper than 3 mm or lesions with metastatic potential, clinical depth dose determinations should be supplemented by instrumentation. Conventionally, this has been done with a thermocouple–pyrometer combination.

An insurance on proper depth dose is accomplished by timing the *halo thaw time* (HTT). This represents the thaw time for the tissue surrounding the target area. For basal cell carcinomas, a HTT of 60 seconds is usually satisfactory; on the nose (because of vascularity and rapid thaw) 45 seconds may be sufficient. This *after the fact* measurement insures that the freezing of the healthy tissue is secondary to deep enlargement of the tissue iceball and not caused by liquid or spray inadvertently applied to the surface of the healthy tissue.

When treating tumors overlying bone or cartilage, fixation of the tumor to these structure during freezing is a useful criterion in determining depth dose. When the tissue becomes fixed, determined by pinching the area surrounding the tumor and trying to move it laterally, it is assumed that the iceball has reached the periosteum or perichondrium (FX or fixation). If freezing is continued (FXFT or fixation freeze time) and the fixation thaw time measured (FXTT or fixation thaw time), the proper depth dose at the surface of the cartilage or bone can be estimated.

TEMPERATURE MEASUREMENT

Because the range of interest is 0C to −60C, pyrometers with a down-side of −75C are the most accurate, but ones with even lower temperature downsides can be used. The most practical size thermocouple-tipped needles are 25-gauge. Thinner needles are too fragile and costly, and thicker ones are unnecessarily gross. A thermocouple-tipped needle gives the operator a single-point temperature reading. The needle is inserted lateral to the tumor and angulated on insertion so that its tip ends up under the center of the tumor and as close to the bottom of the tumor as possible. With freely movable tumors and tumors overlying bone or cartilage, this can be accomplished accurately by palpation alone. If, for research purposes, it is desirable to place the thermocouple at a particular depth, for example, 3 mm beneath the skin surface, it can be done with the aid of a device known as a template. Zacarian designed a template that is commercially available from Frigitronics, Inc., which allows the tip of the thermocouple needle to lie at a predetermined depth. An improvisational method is to attach a clamp to the thermocouple needle so that the tip ends up at a specified depth after insertion (Fig. 4-4). This is particularly useful when using curved needles, which give a more accurate temperature reading as the cold is not transmitted along the shaft.

Thermocouple-tipped needles may also be used to monitor the temperature of the lateral margins of a tumor being frozen. Gage uses a technique in

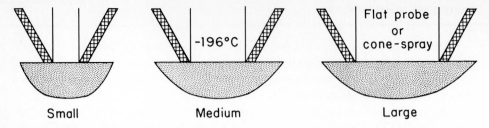

Figure 4-1. Iceball patterns—Flat probes or restricted spray. Depth of freeze = lateral spread of freeze independent of size of cold application area (if cold is applied evenly to target area).

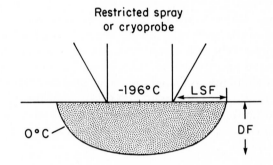

Figure 4-2. Iceball proportions.   Depth of freeze = Lateral spread of freeze

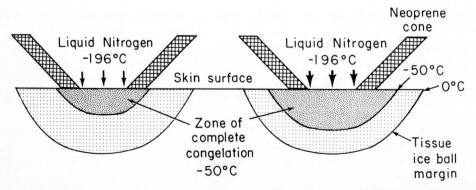

Figure 4-3. Variation in volume of tissue destruction with varying freeze time.

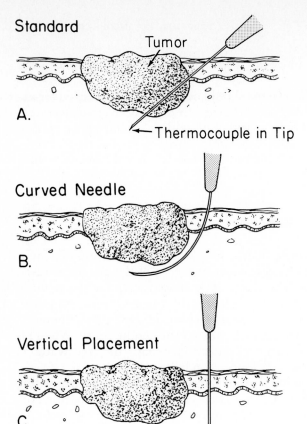

Standard

Tumor

A.

← Thermocouple in Tip

Curved Needle

B.

Vertical Placement

C.

Figure 4-4. Depth dose monitoring thermocouple placement.

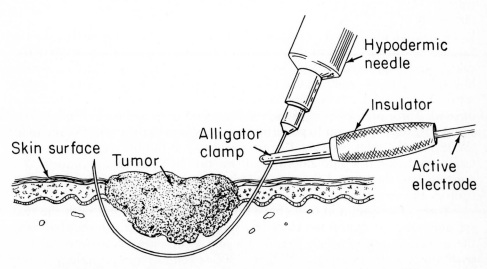

Hypodermic needle

Insulator

Alligator clamp

Active electrode

Skin surface

Tumor

Figure 4-5. Curved electrode placement for use with electrical resistance apparatus.

which the thermocouples are placed at a specified depth at the periphery of a lesion.

Pyrometer–thermocouple systems should be periodically checked for accuracy. The 0 degree calibration can be checked by dipping the thermocouple into an ice–water mixture. Those pyrometers with a −200C range can be checked on the down-side by spraying liquid nitrogen on the tip (−196C). Those with a −75C range can be checked by Fluorocarbon 12 spray (−60C).

ELECTRICAL RESISTANCE MEASUREMENT

An alternate method for judging depth dose is now being evaluated by a number of cryosurgeons. This involves measurement of the electrical resistance in tissue as it is frozen. The electrolytes in extracellular tissue fluid, when in solution, enable conduction of electricity. During the freezing process when individual salts, such as sodium chloride, reach their eutectic point they go out of solution, thereby decreasing the conductivity. When all the electrolytes reach their eutectic point (about −55C) the free water is completely frozen and the tissue no longer conducts electricity.

LePivert of France was the first to develop equipment to measure this parameter in cryosurgery. He measured *impedence* with an alternating current apparatus. Zacarian and Torre separately developed simple direct current apparatus with small batteries that measure tissue resistance. The amount of current used is very small (less than 10 microamp) and meets criteria for human use established by the Food and Drug Administration (FDA). Approval from the FDA for this apparatus has not yet been obtained.

A straight electrode is inserted into the center of the lesion so that the tip extends below the tumor or the electrode can be inserted at the margin of the tumor and angulated so that the tip lies under the center of the tumor. Multiple electrodes may be used and monitored separately or connected in series. Very thin electrodes (for example, 30-gauge hypodermic needles) can be used. Torre prefers using a curved electrode that *cradles* the tumor (Fig. 4-5). A 25-gauge or similar hypodermic needle is bent to the proper shape to fit the lesion and then inserted 1 mm lateral to the tumor, passed under the lesion, and exited 1 mm lateral to it on the far side. This monitors two margins and the base of the tumor. It is also possible to use stainless steel sutures and insert them in various patterns under wide flat lesions.

Torre, Zacarian, and Gage have done comparison studies with the two systems. One can clamp the electrical resistance apparatus to the shaft of a thermocouple-tipped needle to simultaneously compare electrical resistance with temperature readings: −25C to −30C is roughly comparable to 1 megaohm resistance, and −60C to 5 megaohm resistance.

SELECTED READING

Gage A, Carvana J, Garamy G: A comparison of instrument methods of monitoring freezing in cryosurgery. J Dermatol Surg Oncol 9:209, 1983

LePivert P: The measurement of low-frequency electrical impedence as a guide to effective cryosurgery. J Dermatol Surg Oncol 3:395, 1977

Savic M, Zacarian SA: A new impedence-based method for controlled cryosurgery of malignant tumors. J Dermatol Surg Oncol 3:592, 1977

Torre D: Understanding the relationship between lateral spread of freeze and depth of freeze. J Dermatol Surg Oncol 5:51, 1979

Torre D: Correlation of Instruments and Clinical Measurements. Cutaneous Cryosurgery Course. Am Acad Dermatol Annual Meeting, Chicago, Dec. 1983

Torre D: Depth dose in cryosurgery. J Dermatol Surg Oncol 9:219, 1983

Torre D: Cryosurgery of basal cell carcinoma J Am Acad Dermatol 15:917, 1986

GLOSSARY

FT. Freeze Time: Elapsed time from start to end of freeze cycle.

LSF. Lateral Spread of Freeze: Peripheral extension of iceball beyond the area to which cold is applied. With a cryoprobe it is measured from the margin of the probe; with an insulated cone it is measured from the inside margin of the cone; and with the open spray method it is measured from the marked outer margin of the tumor.

DF. Depth of Freeze: Maximun vertical extension of iceball below surface.

CTT. Complete Thaw Time: Elapsed time from stopping cold application until lesion is thawed.

HTT. Halo Thaw Time: Elapsed time from stopping cold application until thaw reaches area where cold was applied (usually to margins of tumors), representing thawing of healthy tissue surrounding tumor.

ITT. Thermocouple Thaw Time: Elapsed time from end of cold application until pyrometer reading is 0C.

FX. Fixation: Refers to adherence of frozen mass (iceball) to underlying bone cartilage.

FXFT. Fixation Freeze Time: Interval time from onset of fixation to end of cold application.

FXTT. Fixation Thaw Time: Interval time from end of cold application until iceball is no longer fixed to underlying bone or cartilage.

TTT. Total Thaw Time: Interval time from end of cold application until entire lesion is completely thawed.

CHAPTER 5

Morbidity and Complications

Morbidity and complications after cryosurgery of benign or malignant lesions are related to the depth and characteristics of the lesion and the depth of freeze used. Because benign lesions do not penetrate as deeply as malignant ones, a lesser amount of freezing is required. The reactions that occur after freezing malignant lesions, on the other hand, are a response of the tissue to deeper freezing and more aggressive treatment. Some reactions can be expected to develop after treatment of any type of lesion, but one should not encounter similar morbidity or complications after treatment of benign lesions as compared with malignant ones.

Morbidity is not a true complication and can be expected to occur to one degree or another after freezing. This depends on the type of lesion, the type of treatment administered, and the specific location treated. It includes edema, exudation, blistering, and pain, which are all early reactions.

The morbidity and complications after cryosurgical treatment can be divided into acute, short- and long-term reactions, and permanent effects.

ACUTE REACTIONS

Edema
After the freezing of benign and malignant lesions, some degree of swelling occurs. The severity of edema is dependent on several factors including the intensity and extent of freezing, the host response to cold, and the location. Urtication, erythema, and edema occur within a few minutes, and the edema

may last for several days. At times, exaggerated edema may occur particularly at the periorbital areas, forehead, mandibular area, and ears (Fig. 5-1). Periorbital edema can be minimized by the use of systemic steroids if no contraindication for its use is present. A short course of corticosteroids is best. Kuflik has recommended 1 cc celestone phosphate 1 M before surgery followed by celestone orally 20 mg per day for 3 days. In addition, the edema can be alleviated with the use of cold water compresses applied frequently. Antihistamines give very little relief.

Pain

Most cryosurgical procedures are relatively painless, as the pain is usually limited by the self-anesthetizing effects of the freezing. This is true for both benign and malignant lesions with some exceptions. In general, a burning sensation during the freezing or thaw period is usual when treating malignant lesions. After the lesion has completely thawed, there is usually no further pain.

Some areas, such as the forehead and temples, are more susceptible to headache. A migraine-type pain can ensue and last for several hours. Use of a mild analgesic will suffice to alleviate this problem.

As for moderate freezing, a throbbing pain can occur after treatment of verruca vulgaris and periungual warts, generally lasting for several hours. Some relief is afforded with cold packs applied to the area immediately after treatment. Mucous membranes are also very sensitive.

Hemorrhage

Hemorrhage is rare, but can occur if a biopsy was performed in conjunction with the cryosurgical procedure. In such instances, it is essential to obtain hemostasis before initiating the cryosurgery.

Nitrogen Gas Insufflation

Nitrogen gas insufflation of subcutaneous tissue is a very rare occurrence, and appears as an immediate swelling around the treated site. This occurs with the open spray method, as nitrogen gas can enter a natural or an iatrogenic opening between the surface and the subcutaneous tissue. The periorbital area is the most likely site for this reaction to occur. It can be prevented by the use of a cryoprobe, a pressure ring, or a cone placed around the open wound before freezing.

Syncope

Syncope is a common reaction during or immediately after treatment of even such benign lesions as verruca vulgaris or periungual warts. It is wise to treat any patient susceptible to syncope in a supine position. This reaction is very rare, however, after treatment of malignant lesions.

SHORT-TERM REACTIONS

Bulla Formation

When treating benign lesions with intact epithelial surfaces, superficial freezing frequently results in production of microscopic or macroscopic bulla. This is due to the separation at the dermal–epidermal junction. It is necessary to obtain this separation for successful treatment of epidermal lesions. Verrucae are a good example. At times, the bullae may become quite large and are often hemorrhagic (Fig. 5-2). When small in size they do not require evacuation and are not painful. Large bullae can cause discomfort and the patient should be instructed to snip the blister with a scissor to release the fluid.

Bullae can also occur after treatment of malignant lesions, particularly at the periphery of the treated area. These resolve within a week and do not interfere with the course of healing.

Infection

Infection is uncommon after cryosurgery, but may develop within a slow healing lesion or underneath a thick crust. Antibiotics are indicated in such cases, after culture of the wound site. Prophylatic antibiotics for cardiac patients with valvular disease may be indicated after deep cryosurgery or cryosurgery combined with biopsy, curettage, or debulking. It is important to mention that the exudation and sloughing that one encounters after deep cryosurgery is to be expected, and does not indicate the presence of secondary infection. This exudative material eventually dries and the site develops a crust.

Delayed Bleeding

Delayed bleeding is an uncommon event, but can occur as the tumor becomes necrotic. A tumor may invade a small vessel that is subsequently frozen. Cryosurgery destroys the cellular elements invading the blood vessel, and the vessel may thus become *unplugged* during the healing stage causing delayed bleeding. When it occurs, it is usually on the cheek, nose, temple, or posterior aspects of the ears. The patient should be instructed to apply pressure for several minutes to the site to stop the bleeding. Additionally, a hemostatic solution can be used along with a gauze dressing. Deodorant products containing aluminum chlorhydrate are usually available to the patient and are good styptics.

Pyogenic Granuloma

Pyogenic granuloma may develop at the treated site several weeks after cryosurgery. This is an uncommon complication. It can be treated by curettage and electrodesiccation or an application of 70 percent aluminum chloride.

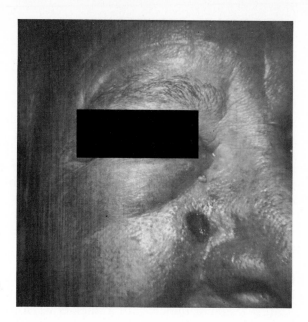

Figure 5-1. Postcryosurgical
periorbital edema.

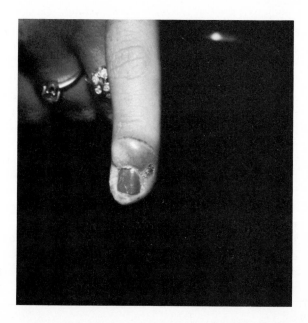

Figure 5-2. Hemorrhagic bulla
after treatment of periungual
wart.

Systemic Reactions

A febrile reaction may develop after cryosurgery, which usually subsides within 24 to 36 hours. This reaction is rare, but may occur in patients who have undergone treatment of large or multiple carcinomas or many large seborrheic keratoses at one sitting. Antipyretics can be used symptomatically.

LONG-TERM REACTIONS

Pseudoepitheliomatous Hyperplasia

A pseudoepitheliomatous hyperplasia can occur 4 to 6 weeks after cryosurgery. This is also an uncommon reaction. Hyperplasia is a self-limited reaction that improves with time. It does not represent a true recurrence and no treatment is necessary.

Nerve Damage

Neuropathy is possible after cryosurgery, but permanent nerve damage is a rare occurrence. Patients may sustain sensory nerve loss of varying degree, and very rarely, motor weakness. Anesthesia and parasthesia are the temporary manifestations of nerve damage, which usually resolve spontaneously over a period of months.

This may develop if a nerve, which lies superficially, is frozen. The areas that require caution include the postauricular area, lateral aspects of fingers, preauricular area, lateral aspect of the tongue, and ulnar fossa of the elbow. Although nerve tissue is sensitive to extreme cold, the neural sheath is rather resistant to freezing; therefore, if the sheath is not deeply frozen, neural regeneration is likely to occur.

Caution should be observed when freezing vulnerable sites; if possible, the lesion to be treated should be manually lifted away from the underlying tissue. Another way to protect the nerve is by injection of sufficient local anesthetic or saline beneath the tumor to lift it, a technique known as ballooning.

Milia

Milia are a complication that is neither serious nor permanent, which can sometimes occur after treatment of a malignant lesion. Milia appear after the site has healed and are located at the periphery. They can be removed simply after piercing with a pointed scapel or blood sample disposable lancet.

PERMANENT EFFECTS

Hypopigmentation

Hypopigmentation commonly occurs after deep freezing and permanent depigmentation is possible. The severity of hypopigmentation is unpredictable;

however, it is more prominent in darker skinned patients and has a predilection for certain areas, such as the tip of the nose, the trunk, and the helix (Fig. 5-3). Patients should be forewarned about the possibility of a whitish area developing at the treated site. This should not be confused with a mild, temporary pigmentary alteration that can be seen after treatment of benign lesions.

Atrophy and Depression

Although scar formation is inevitable after deep cryosurgery, it is usually cosmetically acceptable and the treated sites generally heal smoothly without depression. At times, the skin over the healed site may appear atrophic. This is likely to result if treatment is extended to the subcutaneous tissue (Fig. 5-4). Another type of atrophy can develop on the helix of the ear and the rim of the ala nasi after treatment of large or linear lesions.

Hyperpigmentation

Postinflammatory type hyperpigmentation is not an infrequent occurrence after cryosurgery and is not predictable. This reaction fades gradually but may last up to a year. A typical pigmentary alteration may consist of a central area of hypopigmentation with a surrounding halo of hyperpigmentation (Fig. 5-5). In dark-skinned patients, cryosurgery should be used cautiously.

Hypertrophic Scar

A hypertrophic scar may develop after treatment of a malignancy. It generally forms at the center of the treated site and is slightly raised and reddish. It is usually linear to oval in shape (Fig. 5-6). This reaction is more likely to occur after treatment of large lesions. Hypertrophic scarring is more prevalent on the back, the chest, the forehead, and the temples.

Fortunately, hypertrophic scars usually improve with time and resolve spontaneously. A steroid suspension, such as triamcinolone 5 mg/cc, can be injected intralesionally to aid in the resolution of the scar.

Tissue Defects

Tissue defects, which include notching and perforation, can occur after eradication of cutaneous malignancies. These complications develop on the ears, nose, and eyelids. Notching can occur on the helix, the rim of the ala nasi, the nares, and the margin of the eyelids. It may also be related to the size and depth of the tumor, the depth of freeze, the technique used, and the skill of the physician. Overfreezing is to be avoided if the lesion in question is not a deeply invasive one. Tissue defects, however, may be expected to develop if the tumor has penetrated to the underlying cartilage, if aggressive treatment must be carried out as in the case of large tumors, and at areas prone to notching (Fig. 5-7). Good clinical judgment should be exercised in the selection of cryosurgery for lesions located at these susceptible sites. But if

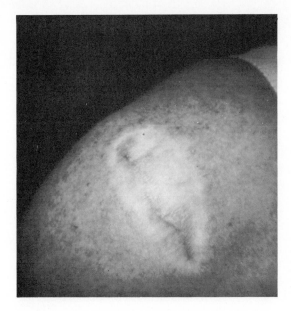

Figure 5-3. Hypopigmentation after treatment of large basal cell carcinoma on shoulder.

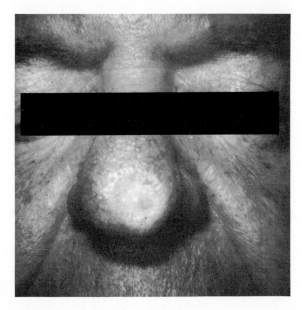

Figure 5-4. Depression resulting after treatment of invasive basal cell carcinoma.

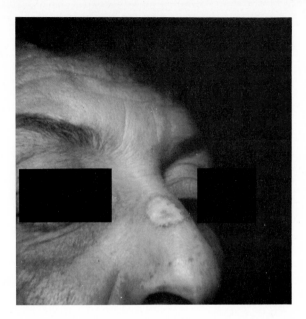

Figure 5-5. Thin ring of hyper-pigmentation at treated site.

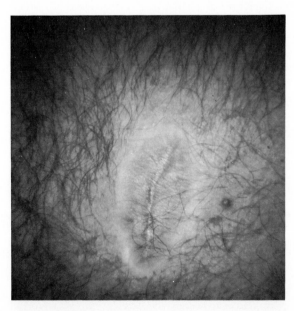

Figure 5-6. Healed chest lesion showing linear hypertrophic scar.

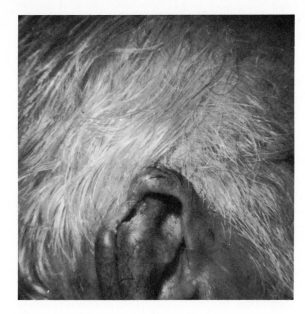

Figure 5-7. Tissue defect at helix after treatment of large basal cell carcinoma.

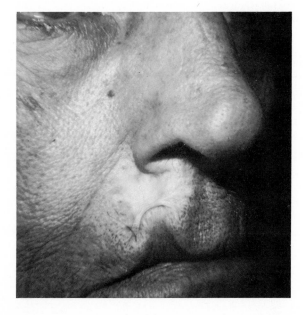

Figure 5-8. Scarring of upper lip after treatment of large tumor.

cryosurgical management is the most suitable choice, then patients should be forewarned about the possibility of some tissue defect.

Scarring

Scarring may be the expected sequelae of treatment of malignant tumors located at certain sites. The locations most likely to be affected include the eyelids, the eyebrow region, the upper lip, and the corners of the mouth. Ectropion of the eyelid is not a common reaction, but can occur if a large tumor at this site is aggressively frozen. Asymmetrical lifting of the eyebrow and the upper lip can result from irregular scarring (Fig. 5-8). Similarly, scarring can cause retraction of the skin at the corners of the mouth resulting in disfigurement. Surgical repair may be indicated in such cases. Extreme caution must be exercised when treating tumors in these areas, and patients must be forewarned of the possibility of a poor cosmetic end result.

Alopecia

Alopecia may be expected to occur if freezing extends to the hair follicles, as is the case of the successful treatment of many malignant lesions. All hair-bearing areas can be affected, including the eyelashes. This complication is commonly seen after treatment of a basal cell carcinoma located on the margin of the eyelid. The development of alopecia after cryosurgery should be fully explained before the treatment.

SELECTED READING

Elton RF: Complication of cutaneous cryosurgery. J Am Acad Dermatol 8:513, 1983

Elton RF: The course of events following cryosurgery. J Dermatol Surg Oncol 3:448, 1977

Kuflik EG, Webb W: Effects of systemic corticosteroids on post-surgical edema and other manifestations of the inflammatory response. J Dermatol Surg Oncol 11:464, 1985

Nix TW Jr: Liquid nitrogen neuropathy. Arch Dermatol 92:185, 1965

Falabella R: Repigmentation of leukoderma by minigrafts of normally pigmented autologous skin. J Dermatol Surg Oncol 4:916, 1978

Suvanprakon P, Dee-Ananlap S, Pongsomboon C: Melanocyte autologus grafting for treatment of leukoderma. J Am Acad Dermatol 13:968, 1985

CHAPTER 6

Treatment of Nonmalignant Lesions

Cryosurgery is now being used by a majority of dermatologists for a wide variety of benign and premalignant lesions. For lesions, such as actinic keratoses, lentigines, or dermatofibromas, it is considered by many to be the treatment of choice. In a variety of conditions, such as mucocele, verrucae, or angiomas, it is an alternate method of therapy that is useful in selected cases. With benign lesions, the cosmetic and functional end results are of major importance, and cure rate is secondary. If insufficient freezing has been administered, it is simple to repeat the treatment at a later date. In some instances cryosurgery can be combined with other modalities, including curettage, to yield better results than the use of cryosurgery alone.

Before using cryosurgery, the cryosurgeon should fully explain to the patient and the family the procedure to be undertaken, the risks involved, and what to expect during cryosurgery and the postoperative period. Patients' questions usually relate to the cost of treatment, the amount of pain they might experience, and whether or not they can continue with their usual activities and employment. Patients' anxieties can be relieved with explanations by the physician and the nurse. The manner and course of treatment, in addition to the healing period, should be explained to the patient. For example, it must be understood that lengthy exudative or crusted stages may prevent the patient from participating in certain social or sports activities, or may cause the patient discomfort at work. It may also be advisable for a family member or companion to accompany the patient home, especially if the lesion is located on or around the eyelids, because edema usually occurs after the treatment.

LOCAL ANESTHESIA

Local infiltration analgesia is seldom necessary when treating superficial lesions, but can be used when desired. In come cases injection of a local anesthetic under a lesion is used to raise it away from underlying tissue (e.g., nerves). Thus, freezing can extend beyond the lesion without harm to healthy tissue that is sensitive to cold. This procedure is termed ballooning.

METHODS OF TREATMENT

There is a wide latitude in the choice of instruments used in treating nonmalignancies. The selection is usually based on one's experience with individual devices and with the variety and frequency of lesions to be treated and the cost.

Nitrous Oxide
Nitrous oxide units can be used in treating nonmalignant lesions, and are useful as stand-by units, and when liquid nitrogen is not readily available.

Dip-Stick Technique
For some lesions, a dip-stick, or swab applicator, can be used with liquid nitrogen. The swab is placed intermittently on the lesion(s) to be treated until the desired amount of freeze is obtained. The most common swab is a readily available cotton-tipped commercial applicator stick (Q-tip). Large swabs sold as vaginal applicators can also be used. Various sized tips may be individually made by twirling cotton around the end of a small dowel. Caution should be taken, especially around vital areas, such as the eyes, to avoid dripping of liquid nitrogen from the swab.

Liquid Nitrogen Apparatus
A liquid nitrogen unit is the apparatus of choice because it is most versatile. Liquid nitrogen is capable of treating malignant lesions as well as superficial or deep benign tumors. Either hand-held, table top, or floor model units are effective, and are adaptable for spray or probe use.

Open Spray
In treating nonmalignant lesions with liquid nitrogen spray, clinical criteria are used to estimate proper depth and extent of freezing. Two of the more valuable criteria are lateral spread of freeze and thaw time. The spray is

Spiral

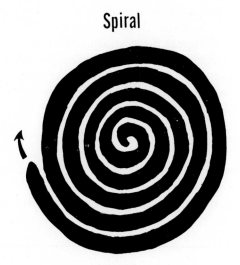

Paint Brush

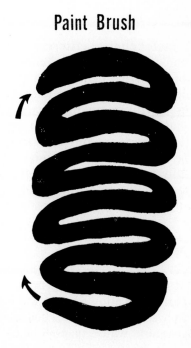

Figure 6-1. Spray patterns.

directed at the lesion to be treated so that it is evenly frozen. Intermittent application may be necessary to avoid freezing too deeply. With large lesions, a paint brush or spiral pattern can be used (Fig. 6-1). The goal in treating nonmalignant lesions is to completely freeze the lesion, a very small rim of healthy tissue peripheral to the lesion, and a thin layer of healthy tissue deep to the lesion. A properly frozen lesion will be entirely white and hard on palpation. A *halo* of frozen healthy tissue will appear peripheral to the lesion. The halo should be even and varies from 1 mm to 3.5 mm depending on the type of lesion being treated (benign or premalignant). This halo represents the lateral spread of freeze from the area frozen as the liquid nitrogen should be applied only to the lesion. With practice, this can easily be performed with the open-spray technique.

Confined Spray
When learning cryosurgery use of a lateral limiting device to confine the spray is helpful. Otoscope cones with openings of 2, 3, 5, 7 mm are satisfactory. Containment of the spray allows for more accurate assessment of the halo lateral spread of freeze.

Cryoprobe
A lateral spread of freeze is also easily observed with a flat cryoprobe.

THAW TIME

A useful clinical criteria for estimating proper depth of freezing is observation of thawing of lesion. An evenly treated lesion will thaw evenly. With uneven treatment the area receiving less freezing will thaw faster. The deeper the freeze, the longer the thaw. The thaw time of the lesion itself is used with nonmalignancies and is termed the total thaw time (TTT). The thaw time of the surrounding healthy tissue is called the halo thaw time (HTT) and is more widely used when treating malignant lesions but can also be used with thicker benign or premalignant lesions. This is discussed more fully in Chapter 7. Table 6-1 gives treatment guidelines for nonmalignant lesions, the total thaw time, and the radius of the lateral of freeze (halo) suggested for various lesions.

AFTERCARE

Aftercare for cryosurgery of nonmalignancies is relatively simple. Normal bathing is allowed, and the lesions are washed daily with a cleansing solution such as aqueous benzalconium chloride, hydrogen peroxide, alcohol, soap and water, or povidone–iodine. Topical antibiotics are advised only if

seconds, or application of liquid nitrogen with a cotton swab is used until the lesion is slightly blanched white. The spray is better to use than the cryoprobe.

3. Cysts. Some firm cysts are best treated by intralesional steroids, but soft fluctuant cysts or cysts covered by eschar can be treated by spraying liquid nitrogen for several seconds until blanching indicates the end point of treatment. Occasionally, a longer freeze, 10 to 15 seconds, are necessary for resistant or recalcitrant cysts, particularly those on the back. Multiple cysts may be treated in this way.

Cryotherapy can also be useful in treating certain patients taking isotretinoin (Accutane), who sometimes experience flare ups of lesions between the first and third months of therapy. These cysts can sometimes clear in 5 to 7 days after cryotherapy.

Acne Scarring

The technique for acne scarring differs considerably from that used in the treatment of individual lesions. Careful consideration must be given to skin type, pigmentation, epidermal thickness, and location of the scarring. Cryotherapy is most effective for circinate superficial scars, some hypertrophic scars, and some keloids.

Technique

1. Skin is sectioned off in six to nine rectangles on each cheek, approximately 2 by 4 cm each, using a skin marking pencil or gentian violet. The patient sits upright. Premedication is usually not necessary.
2. The eyes are protected by goggles, and a plastic raincoat or similar item, is draped on the patient in case of any dripping of liquid nitrogen during the procedure.
3. Each rectangle on the cheek is spray frozen for approximately 5 to 15 seconds, using the special spray slit-tip accessory, if it is available. The spray slit-tip accessory is available with many hand-held units. Longer freezing times of 20 or more seconds may be required to treat more hypertrophic or keloidal scars. Occasionally, cryoprobes may be used for these types of scars.
4. The liquid nitrogen is applied in a painting or shaving motion moving up and down the cheek. Freezing longer than 15 to 20 seconds is usually not recommended as excessive freezing of the skin could result in atrophy or permanent loss of pigmentation.
5. In thin-skinned areas, as under the eyes, on the neck, and over the mandible, no more than 5 to 8 seconds of freezing is suggested.
6. If the patient experiences more than moderate stinging and burning, a short period may be required after several areas have been treated.

This also allows time for dissemination of the vapor, which may obstruct vision if it clouds the treatment field. Also, excess moisture on the spray can be shaken or wiped off to prevent dripping of liquid nitrogen onto the patient.

Usually no postoperative medication is necessary. During the crusting phase, every effort is made to avoid premature removal of the crust. Premature removal of the crust could delay healing and affect cosmetic end results. It also increases the risk of secondary infection. Mild, temporary hypopigmentation resulting from peeling usually occurs. Routine topical acne medications are usually discontinued for at least a week. Patients are also advised to avoid sun exposure for at least 6 weeks. Sunscreens may be used when sun exposure is unavoidable. Cosmetic foundation bases are available that are formulated with sunscreens to obscure the erythema and protect against possible sun damage.

Acne-Related Conditions

Acne Keloidalis
Papules and plaques of acne keloidalis may be flattened considerably with 20 to 40 seconds of spray freezing with an intermediate spray nozzle opening. Thicker, more nodular lesions may be treated with the combination of intralesional steriods and freezing. In other cases, the extensive plaques can be removed first by shave excision and then freezing the base.

Acne Rosacea
The papules, pustules, and telangiectasis of rosacea have been improved in some cases by liquid nitrogen spray. Papules and pustules are treated the same as described previously. When treating rhinophyma, a freeze time of 60 seconds is usually necessary to reduce hyperplastic tissue in this condition.

Cryotherapy may also be used in conjunction with other procedures such as dermabrasion or collagen implants. Sometimes freezing alone is used for several weeks before dermabrasion, and may serve to lessen the amount of cysts on the face, making dermabrasion easier to perform. Because permanent pigmentary alteration can develop with repeated freezing, dermabrasion should be considered for those patients who do not show significant improvement of their scarring after at least two to three freezing treatments, especially for those with deeper irregular scars.

When collagen is used, freezing should probably precede the implants. It is not known at this point whether freezing would add or detract from the collagen procedure, if used after the implants.

Edema of the face, sometimes moderate to severe, can occur. This is especially true around the periorbital areas.

Pigmentary changes can also be seen, even with superficial freezing of 10 to 15 seconds; although uncommon, Graham has observed pigmentary changes in at least three patients. This pigmentation faded within 2 to 6 months. Hypopigmentation is usually transitory, and has not been permanent in most cases. In dark-skinned patients, hypopigmentation that occurs usually repigments within a few months. However, all dark-skinned individuals should be treated with due caution and warnings.

Angiomas and Other Vascular Tumors

Certain angiomas and other vascular tumors can respond well to cryosurgical techniques. Much of our knowledge concerning hemangiomas has come from the work of Dr. Castro-Ron of Caracas.

Immature hemangiomas can respond well, but only lesions that have reason to be treated should be frozen as many of these resolve spontaneously. Lesions selected are usually those that show rapid growth or that interfere with a bodily orifice or function (Fig. 6-2).

The so-called cavernous hemangioma are those lesions that have large, irregular endothelial-lined spaces and that are situated deep in the subcutaneous tissue. Cryosurgery, for the cavernous hemangiomas that are not very deep, is an excellent therapeutic modality. Cryosurgery is particularly useful where other more aggressive methods have failed. This is especially true in lesions in the oral cavity.

Treatment Technique

1. Local or regional anesthesia may or may not be used depending on the size and location of the lesion. For instance, lesions in the anterior and middle third of the mouth require local or regional anesthesia, whereas general anesthesia and tracheostomy are required for lesions located at the posterior third of the mouth and the oropharynx.
2. Osler-Rendu-Weber and angiokeratoma lesions respond well and are managed by placing a pointed cryoprobe in the center of each lesion. Freezing is carried out for several seconds until the entire lesion is frozen and a 1-mm halo of frozen healthy tissue appears around the lesion.

Lymphangiomas

Lymphangiomas, because of their ill-defined boundaries and extent, represent a difficult task for excisional surgery or other therapeutic modalities. Cryosurgery is an alternate method of alleviating the annoying symptoms of the superficial components, such as the verrucose appearance, the serous or serosanguinous exudate after minor trauma, and subsequent lymphangitis resulting from superimposed infection. Many patients who have lymphangiomas of the tongue, trunk, or residual lesions around scars left from surgi-

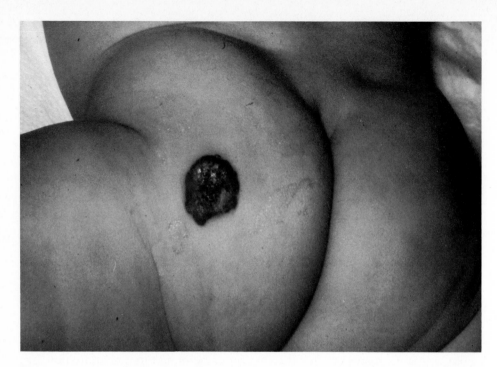

Figure 6-2. Angioma. **A.** Angioma of the buttock.

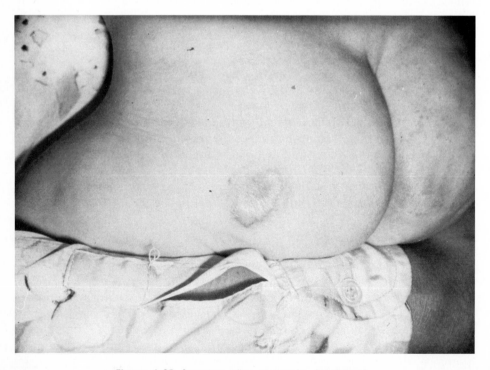

Figure 6-2B. Scarring after cryoprobe treatment.

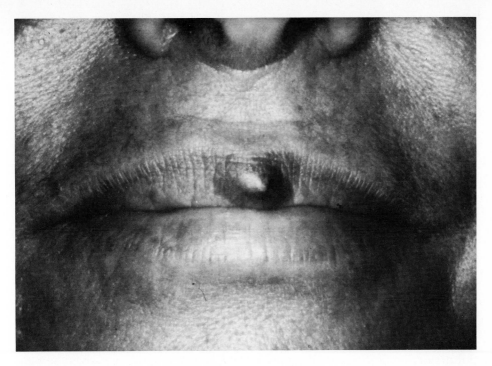

Figure 6-2C. Venous lake of lip.

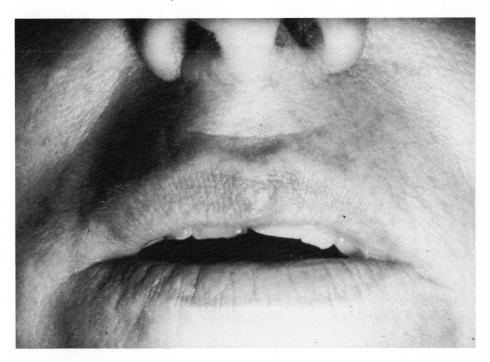

Figure 6-2D. Postoperative results. (Figs. 6-2**A** through 6-2**D** courtesy of Dr. Gilberto Castro-Ron.)

cally excised tumors, have been controlled and eventually cured by repeated applications of the cyroprobe to the superficial elements.

Treatment is carried out by selecting a flat probe that fits the size of the lesion as closely as possible. The cryoprobe is prechilled and is applied firmly at multiple sites at a single sitting until a 1- to 2-mm rim of frozen halo is noted around the probe or to the outside of the lesion. Repeat treatments may be necessary at approximately 8- to 10-week intervals.

Venous Lakes

Some physicians do not consider venous lakes to be true hemangiomas, but rather simple venous dilatations, occasionally of traumatic origin. For treatment, a cryoprobe technique is used. Usually no anesthesia is required. A flat or round probe is selected with a diameter either of the same size or slightly smaller than that of the lesion to be treated. The probe is prechilled and is applied with firm pressure to the center of the lesion to squeeze out the blood content. Freezing is continued until a halo of 1 to 1.5 mm is seen around the probe or to the outside of the lesion. The probe is removed when the halo is attained. If the venous lake is located on the lips, the ice front should not be allowed to extend beyond the vermilion border as this can result in cicatricial distortion of the area. Postoperatively, small- to moderate-sized hemangiomas, including those of the oral cavity and tongue, heal without undue complications or morbidity (Figs. 6-2C and 6-2D). There is minimal loss of healthy tissue and scarring. Minor symptoms, such as edema and salivation when working around the mouth, can occur for several days. Freezing large masses of hemangiomas, however, can present with increased morbidity over that seen with cryosurgical procedures performed on other benign lesions. Due to heavy vascularization of hemangiomas, treatment with cryosurgery must sometimes be more aggressive and more vigorous than with treatment of other benign lesions and even of certain malignancies. One must be prepared, therefore, to deal with certain undesirable postoperative reactions that are basically accentuations of those seen with less potent freezing.

Notably, massive edema can occur in the frozen and adjacent healthy tissues. Edema can last for 10 to 15 days and may be associated with excessive and annoying salivation when lesions of the mouth are treated. Interference with swallowing and respiration have also been known to occur. Particularly in and around the mouth, the treated areas become malodorous and necrotic. The use of a soothing mouthwash is helpful during these periods. In some cases, nutrition by nasal gastric tube or by the parental route is necessary for several days after freezing. A prophylactic tracheostomy should be performed if treatment is in the posterior part of the oral cavity. Swelling of the tongue is sometimes so great that it may protrude from the mouth.

Healing time for treated angiomas varies according to the size and the location of the lesion. If the tumor is small and located on the face, it may require up to 3 to 4 weeks or longer to heal. If it is located on the scalp or of a larger size, it may take more than 6 to 8 weeks to heal. Repeat freezing should be carried out after the scab has fallen away. This will usually occur after 6 to 10 weeks, but it may take longer.

It should be noted that bleeding is actually an unusual event after treating hemangiomas. Hemorrhage has been observed immediately or several days after cryosurgery, which could be a result of trauma. Rarely, late hemorrhage that develops 1 to 2 weeks after cryosurgery, has been observed as necrotic tissue sloughs away. In these cases, suture ligation or electrocoagulation of the vessels under local anesthetic may be necessary.

Carbuncle

Cryosurgery for carbuncles can be considered as adjunctive therapy only. It is certainly not advocated for all lesions. The indication for treatment would be about the same as one would consider if electrodessication or curettage were to be used. A spray technique is primarily used. After opening the lesion the spray is centered into the cavity and continued until the walls are frozen. A small, rounded probe can also be used. One should be careful that the pressure from the spray does not splatter the contents of the carbuncle.

Chondrodermatitis

Controversy still surrounds the treatment of chondrodermatitis by cryosurgery. Sometimes equivocal results are obtained, and excisional surgery might still be necessary. On occasion, one also finds that lesion of chondrodermatitis is actually stimulated or irritated by cryosurgery. Indeed, many lesions can be treated with a solid freeze to the area. A total thaw time of 45 to 60 seconds is usually adequate. Intralesional steroids can also be injected before or after the procedure. More than one treatment may be necessary and this is usually carried out at intervals of 4 to 8 weeks.

Dermatofibroma

Dermatofibroma can be a management problem. If scalpel excision is used, an oval atrophic scar frequently ensues giving a poor cosmetic result in many instances, especially if the lesion is located on the lower extremities or back. Cryosurgery is the treatment of choice (Fig. 6-3). An open-spray technique can be used particularly on larger lesions. After the central portion of the lesion is removed by punch biopsy and hemostasis is obtained, the spray is centered into the biopsy site and continued until a 1- to 2-mm frozen halo appears around the lesion.

A cryoprobe or spray contained by a otoscope cone, however, can be effectively used in the majority of lesions with a flat or slightly elevated lesion. A saucerizing shave excision biopsy with a scalpel may be done before freezing. This leaves a shallow concave surface. Hemostasis is obtained by application of 70 percent aluminum chloride solution. A flat-head type cryoprobe or cone with an opening usually one-half to two-thirds the diameter of

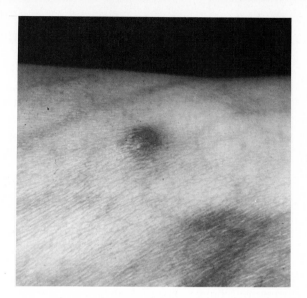

Figure 6-3. Dermatofibroma.
A. Dermatofibroma of the thigh.

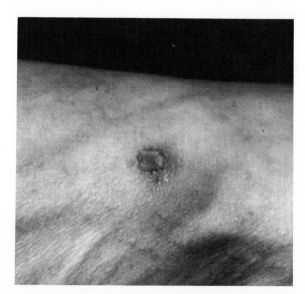

Figure 6-3B. Exophytic portion
excised (saucerization) for biopsy and hemostases obtained
by application of 70 percent
aluminum chloride.

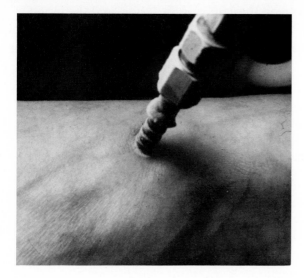

Figure 6-3C. Cryoprobe technique being used.

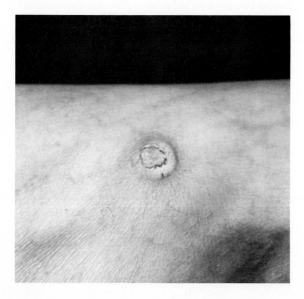

Figure 6-3D. Lesion at completion of freeze.

the lesion is selected. It is placed on the center of the lesion, and the lesion is then frozen until a small 1- to 2-mm frozen halo forms around the tumor. The depth of freeze is thus measured by the lateral spread of freeze (LSF) rather than thaw time.

Granuloma Pyogenicum

Because granuloma pyogenicum lesions are vascular, they may not respond consistently. Cryosurgery, however, can be of benefit in some cases. Small lesions are spray frozen, whereas larger lesions may require a cryoprobe. In either event, the lesion is frozen solidly until a 1- to 2-mm frozen halo appears around the base of the lesion. Retreatments may be necessary. It should be remembered that for these and other vascular lesions, a harder than anticipated freeze may be necessary. If there is any question about the diagnosis, the lesion may be curetted off for biopsy, the base electrocoagulated, and then sprayed with liquid nitrogen to yield a thaw time of 15 to 30 seconds.

Hidradenitis Suppurativa

Small, localized hidradenitis suppurativa lesions may be treated by solid freezing of the surface of the lesion by spray or probe. Extensive lesions are best treated by marsupializing the tunnels, curetting the tunnel linings, applying 70 percent aluminum chloride for hemostasis, and then spray freezing the lining.

Keloids

Keloids respond variably to cryosurgery. There are several ways to treat these lesions. Usually a small lesion can be frozen solid. A large lesion might be treated by excising nine-tenths of the lesion, leaving a thin shell of keloid, and then freezing this shell. The use of intralesional steriods, however, probably increases favorable results. Steroids can be injected either prefreezing or postfreezing. Spray technique is used most commonly, but a solid freeze is usually obtained in any method. Most young keloids respond well. Whatever the method used and whatever the age of the keloid, however, multiple treatments are usually required.

Keratoacanthoma

Most dermatologists wish to submit keratoacanthoma lesions to the pathologist for confirmation of diagnosis, therefore, cryosurgery is usually an adjunctive treatment to the base after the lesion has been removed by curettage or excisional biopsy. The base is then frozen solidly after hemostasis is obtained. A frozen halo of healthy tissue of at least 3 mm is recommended. Cryosurgery alone can be used in those smaller multiple lesions.

Keratosis (Actinic)

Actinic keratoses are the ideal target for cryosurgery. Cotton swabs dipped in liquid nitrogen can be effectively used. The open-spray technique is superior and allows many lesions to be treated effectively in a very short time. The spray is directed onto the surface of the keratosis until the surface becomes white and hard and a 1- to 2-mm halo of healthy tissue surrounding the lesion becomes white. Thaw time is usually 10 to 15 seconds, but thicker lesions can be treated for a thaw time of 20 to 30 seconds. A cure rate of 95 to 98 percent can be expected by experienced operators.

Keratosis (Seborrheic)

The thickness and number of lesions present help determine the techniques used. The thin-type seborrheic keratoses can be treated like actinic keratoses by application of a spray of short duration (Fig. 6-4). For thicker lesions to be treated by a spray alone, prolonged spraying is necessary, which demands more experience and judgment to assess proper depth of freeze and also causes much more surrounding hyperpigmentation on healing. An alternative technique is frequently used for these thicker lesions.

The lesion is sprayed superficially just enough to make the raised portion firm but not solidly frozen. The lesion is then curetted to strip off the raised portion from the surface of the skin. Once this is done, a hemostatic solution is applied to the surface. A covering dressing strip completes the process. If desired Gel Foam in the form of dental pack or powder can be applied under the dressing to assure a dry wound. This technique can also be used on flat lesions and usually minimizes postinflammatory hyperpigmentation. Multiple lesions can be treated in a single visit, and excellent cosmetic results are usually obtained.

Lentigo

There is no perfect procedure for treatment of lentigo. The results produced with cryosurgery, however, certainly justify its consideration for use in many cases. Large senile lentigines respond well to a single spray treatment. When multiple small lentigines are treated, all of the color may not be removed in one treatment. Repeat, light treatments may be needed and given at 3- to 6-week intervals. Spray or probe techniques may be used. With the spray, a small diameter tip is used to spray the lesion so that a total thaw time of 10 to 20 seconds is obtained. When using a probe, a flat-head type slightly smaller than the lesion is placed in the center. Freezing is then carried just to 1 mm beyond the lesion margin. When treating multiple lesions, only a few should be treated for testing purposes at the first visit. Also, when treating the large type, a central clearing with a darker peripheral rim of pigmentation at the border or slightly outside of the lesion sometimes occurs. This can take weeks to months to resolve.

Leukoplakia

Leukoplakia of the lip, tongue, and buccal mucosa also responds well to cryosurgical methods (Fig. 6-5). On the lip, after a biopsy is obtained, a spray technique is used. The lesion is usually sprayed frozen by a vertical or horizontal paint brush pattern. When the entire lip needs to be frozen, it is

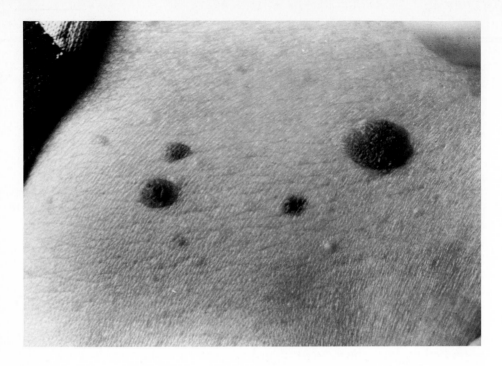

Figure 6-4. Seborrheic keratoses. **A.** Preoperative.

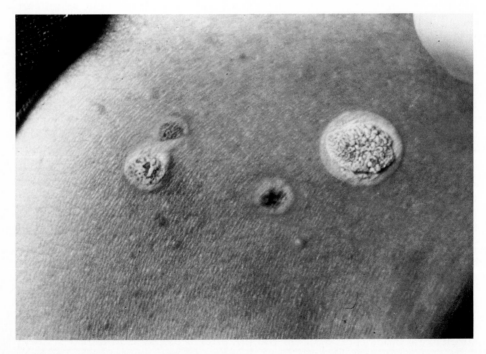

Figure 6-4B. After spray freezing, note halo of frozen tissue extending beyond lesions.

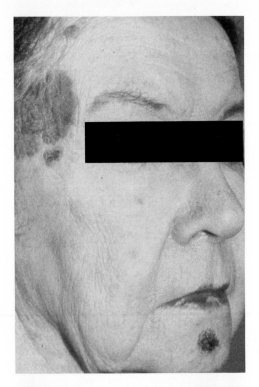

Figure 6-4C. Multiple keratoses of the face.

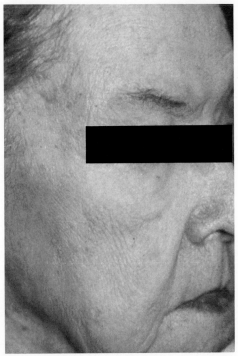

Figure 6-4D. Postoperative results.

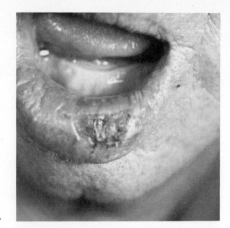

Figure 6-5. Leukoplakia.
A. Ulcerative leukoplakia of the lip.

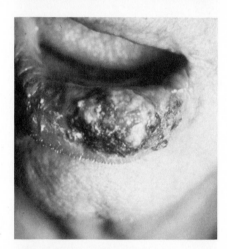

Figure 6-5B. Crusting after cryosurgery.

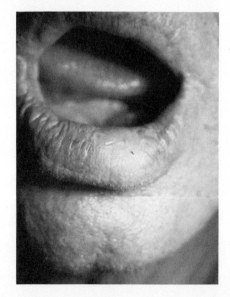

Figure 6-5C. Final result.

optional but probably desirable to freeze no more than one-half of the lip in any one session thus giving the patient less discomfort. This also allows for more comfortable eating and drinking during the healing phase. Total thaw times for the lip are usually 1 to 1.5 minutes. Thick crusting can, and usually does, occur on the lip after a few days to a week. Usually hydrogen peroxide washes to gently remove excessive crusts after the first week are all that is necessary to keep the area clean and to provide good healing. On the buccal mucosa and the tongue, large areas can be eradicated. Either the spray or the probe technique can be used for this. When using a cryoprobe in the mouth, however, it should be remembered that, to keep the probe from sticking to the buccal mucosa, prechilling of the probe and moving it around on the target help prevent this. Open-end probe devices are useful in this application. When treating the tongue, particularly on the lateral posterior aspect, scarring or nerve loss has been reported. In addition, when using the spray, vapors can be a problem. A suction apparatus can help relieve this.

Molluscum Contagiosum

When treating molluscum lesions, a pointed probe or an otoscope cone with a small opening to contain the spray is useful. The elevated portion of the lesion is frozen until a barely visible white rim appears around the base. An alternate method is to use a fluorinated hydrocarbon spray. The lesions are usually sprayed very superficially in groups. A small curette or cuticle knife (V cutter) is then used to evacuate the central portion of the molluscum. This usually results in cure, is not painful to the patient, and multiple lesions can be treated in this manner.

Mucocele

Mucoceles respond favorably to cryosurgery (Fig. 6-6). Dermatologists are increasingly using cryosurgery as an alternate treatment for these benign tumors. Mucoceles of the lip can be frozen solidly with slight pressure until a normal frozen rim occurs outside the border of the lesion. Repeat treatments may be necessary at about 8-week intervals. To our knowledge, no one has a large series of mucoceles, and thus we cannot state that cryosurgery is unequivocally the treatment of choice. It can be stated, however, that cryosurgery is an alternate treatment of choice in many cases. Again, one should note that chilling the cryoprobe before application and moving it around slightly on the target surface can help prevent sticking to the mucous membrane. Some dermatologists prefer to evacuate the contents of the cyst before treatment and some prefer to marsupialize the lesion and spray freeze the base.

Porokeratosis Plantaris Discreta

Excellent responses to cryosurgery have been shown to occur in treatment of porokeratosis plantaris discreta. The method calls for a local anesthetic after which the surface of the lesion is pared before the initial spray freeze. After a

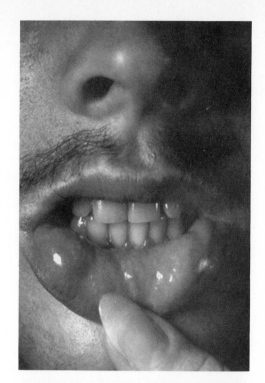

Figure 6-6. Mucocele. **A.** Preoperative.

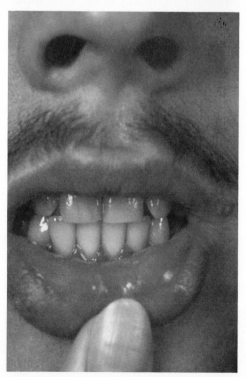

Figure 6-6B. Healed results.

relatively solid spray freeze, debridement of each lesion is carried out at 2-week intervals. At these visits, any residual core is frozen. Several treatments are usually necessary for expected results.

Sebaceous Hyperplasia

Sebaceous hyperplasia are primarily cosmetic and, therefore, pose a double problem; the need for effective eradication and minimal to no scarring. Cryosurgery is well suited to this end. A cryoprobe technique is used. A fine pointed probe is placed into or on the punctum of the lesions with a 3- to 8-second freeze usually being sufficient. The yellowish buds seem to blanche, and a very small rim (1 mm) of healthy tissue is also frozen. Once this is done, it is not necessary to time the thaw. Many lesions can be treated at a single sitting, but retreatments are needed and are carried out at around 4- to 8-week intervals. Results are probably comparable to fine needle electrodessication.

Steatocystoma Multiplex

Several patients with soft cysts (steatocystoma multiplex) have multiple lesions treated by 30 to 60 seconds of liquid nitrogen spray. The lesions become suppurative and drain after several days. They heal with a dilated pore. Because of the multitude of lesions in this condition, patients find freezing more acceptable than excision of the cysts.

Trichiasis

Cryosurgery is being used extensively by dermatologists and ophthalmologists for treatment of trichiasis. After shielding the globe with a sterile insulating device, such as a retractor, a fine spray technique or small pointed probe is used. Instrument monitoring may indeed be necessary for optimal treatment of these lesions. A 25-gauge or finer thermocouple-tipped needle is inserted near the base of the follicle and horizontal to the lid. The area to be treated is then frozen to a temperature of about $-15C$. When this temperature is reached the procedure is terminated. Two freeze cycles are sometimes used. If electrical resistance apparatus is used, epilation needles are inserted in the follicle and 1 megaohm is the target resistance. More than one treatment may be necessary for eradication and effective control of these ingrowing hairs. Although both lids can be treated, the upper lids do not respond as well as do the lower.

Verruca

Verrucae respond not only by type but by location of the lesions (Fig. 6-7). Digitate lesions probably respond best. A spray technique is used for these and most other warts; the entire lesion is frozen with a slight amount of base and surrounding rim. Thaw times are usually not necessary.

Periungual verrucae respond well but are sometimes refractory to treatment with cryosurgery. Probably a swab is best or fine spray from one of the

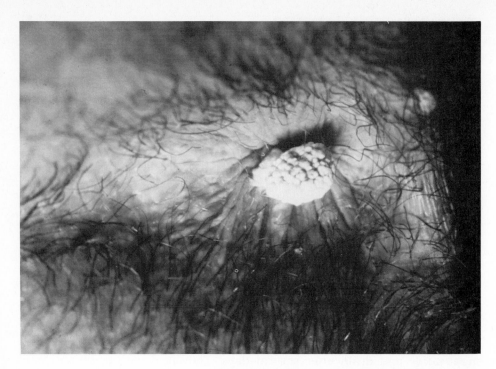

Figure 6-7. Verrucae. **A.** Condylomata of the anus after spray freezing.

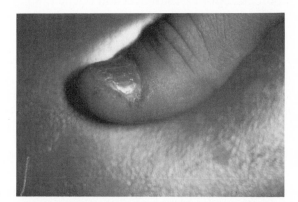

Figure 6-7B. Periungual wart.

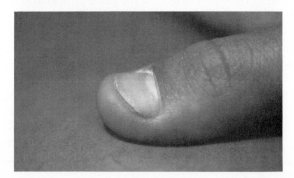

Figure 6-7C. Result after spray freezing.

small portable hand-held units. One should be careful when treating these in that undue pain is sometimes seen, and freezing the nail plate should be avoided.

For verruca vulgaris on glabrous skin, a swab or again use of a small portable hand-held unit is probably best. Small children are less frightened by application of a Q-tip. A spray is used if an instrument system is employed. With small lesions it is best to control the spread of freeze with control devices such as otoscope cones.

To eradicate verruca plana either a superficial spray to the area, small probes, or small opening otoscope cones are used for individual lesions. The technique, however, is rather slow.

Plantar and palmar verruca can be treated with a process similar to that described in porokeratosis plantaris discreta. Local anesthetics may or may not be needed. Cryosurgery alone for these lesions is not encouraging as the recurrence rate is high. Various authors report good results with combined techniques.

Condylomata acuminatum can respond favorably to cryosurgery. Multiple digitate lesions respond best. The technique is similar to that described for digitate verrucae. Thaw times are usually not necessary. Often cryosurgery is used in combination with podophyllin. For this technique the warts are first sprayed slightly with liquid nitrogen, then 25 percent podophyllin in tincture of benzoin is applied. This is repeated at 1- to 2-week intervals. This technique should be considered in cases where podophyllin alone fails.

Miscellaneous

There are several conditions or tumors that have been shown to respond to cryosurgical techniques, but for which a great deal of experience has not yet been gained. Some will be mentioned here for completeness.

One case of cure has been reported for a localized chromoblastomycosis near and above the lip. A spray technique was used with a solid freeze. A total thaw time of 3 to 4 minutes was used, and repeat treatments were necessary to obtain cure.

Results in a small series of swimming pool granuloma have also been reported. The technique was to remove the lesion and then freeze the base.

SELECTED READING

Graham GF: Cryosurgery in the treatment of acne. In Epstein E, Epstein E Jr (eds): Skin Surgery. Springfield, Ill., Charles C. Thomas, 1982, p. 889

Hill AC, Dougherty JW, Torre D: Cryosurgical treatment of dermatofibromas. Cutis 16(3):507, 1975

Kuflik EG: Cryosurgical treatment of periungual warts. J Dermatol Surg Oncol 10:673, 1984

Lubritz RR: Cryosurgical spray patterns. J Dermatol Surg Oncol 4:138, 1978

Lubritz RR, Smolewski SA: Cryosurgery cure rate of premalignant leukoplakia of the lower lip. J Dermatol Surg Oncol 9:235, 1983

Lubritz RR, Smolewski SA: Cryosurgery cure rate of actinic keratoses. J Am Acad Dermatol 7:631, 1982

Lubritz RR, Torre D: Cutaneous cryosurgery for nonmalignant and malignant lesions. In Coleman WP, Colon GA, Davis RS (eds): Outpatient Surgery of the Skin. New Hyde Park, N.Y., Medical examination, 1983, p 188

Sullivan J, Beard C, Bullock J: Cryosurgery for treatment of trichiasis. Am Ophthalmol 82(1): 117, 1976

Torre D, Lubritz RR: Cutaneous cryosurgery: Treatment of nonmalignant lesions. (Clinical Courses in Dermatology No.2), American Academy of Dermatology, 1976

CHAPTER 7

Treatment of Malignant Lesions

Cryosurgery is a relatively simple and effective form of treatment for cutaneous neoplasms and the cure rate is high. At the present time, it is not indicated as primary treatment of malignant melanoma. Cryosurgery can be used for small, medium, or large lesions, for selected recurrent lesions, and for lesions that present problems in management by other modalities. It should be emphasized that only lesions that have definable borders are candidates for cryosurgical treatment. The primary goal of treatment of malignant lesions is thorough eradication of the tumor, with preservation of as much of the healthy tissue as possible. Good cosmetic result is a secondary goal.

This chapter is intended for physicians who are familiar with cutaneous tumors, and who wish to add cryosurgery to their therapeutic armamentarium.

Before undertaking cryosurgical treatment of skin cancers one must determine which lesions are good candidates for this method. Also, the clinician must have an understanding of the cryobiologic effects of deep freezing, the operation of cryosurgical equipment, and the morbidity and risks associated with cryosurgery. The reader is, therefore, advised to become familiar with the information in the preceding chapters before attempting to treat malignant lesions.

INDICATIONS AND CONTRAINDICTIONS

Because cryosurgery is a field therapy, similar to roentgen–ray therapy, the margins of the tumor should be known before treatment. Only those tumors that can be clearly delineated should be treated by cryosurgery. With most skin cancers, the horizontal margins and tumor depth can be determined by observation, palpation, and ballottement. Pinching the skin lateral and medial to the tumor can sometimes be helpful in recognizing the tumor margin. Moving the tumor over underlying bone or cartilage to determine possible fixation of the tumor to such a structure is also helpful. With tumors not fixed to bone or cartilage, these anatomic structures can be used to judge the depth of the tumor. Chemical delineation is sometimes helpful; application of 5-fluorouracil for a week or 10 days before cryosurgery can be used. Curettage is another good method of delineating tumors. Some tumors, such as sclerosing basal cell carcinomas, do not curette well and have margins that are difficult to determine clinically. Multiple, small punch biopsies at the periphery of the tumor are sometimes sufficient; but if this type of tumor cannot be delineated, some method other than cryosurgery should be used.

Any tumor whose margins cannot be determined should be considered a contraindication for cryosurgery. Malignancies extending into the inner canthus, those deep in the nasolabial fold, or recurrent lesions with scar tissue are a relative contraindication. Cryosurgery is also contraindicated in patients with severe cold intolerance, such as cryoglobulinemia, cryofibrogenemia, cold urticaria, and autoimmune diseases.

For some lesions cryosurgery is particularly indicated. This group includes large superficial basal cell carcinomas overlying bone or cartilage and for lesions in areas as the anterior chest where hypertrophic scarring is frequent. Another indication for cryosurgery is palliation of inoperable lesions; pain can be lessened, odor eliminated, and friable bleeding masses destroyed. Poor risk or debilitated patients, those with pacemakers or on anticoagulant therapy can also be treated by cryosurgery. Allergy to local anesthetics is not a contraindication as patients can be treated with no analgesia or after the use of cold normal saline injected around and under the lesion.

CRYOSURGERY FOR MALIGNANT LESIONS

Documentation
The physician should record the patient's history, duration, description, location, size of the lesion, and any previous treatment given. This information is entered into the patient's medical record, and, if one wishes, it can be recorded on a separate card and retained in a file exclusively for cryosurgery of malignant lesions.

Visual documentation is easily obtained by taking before, during, and after photographs of the lesion and treated site. With proper photographic equipment, good close-up shots will provide a permanent record of the results of cryosurgery.

Explanation and Consent
The procedure, risk, course, and expected results should be fully explained to the patient and consent obtained.

Preparation for Cryosurgery

Before the actual freezing of the lesion the patient must be prepared and the cryosurgical equipment and accessories made ready. The cryosurgical device should be filled with liquid nitrogen beforehand, and sterile thermocouple needles should be connected to the pyrometer. A selection of spray tip accessories, cones, or cryoprobes should be at hand. Premedication is not usually necessary, nor is general anesthesia required. Except for treatment of extensive superficial basal cell epithelioma, 1 to 2 percent lidocaine is usually injected locally to alleviate discomfort. Injection of larger quantities of anesthetic agent or supplemental saline solution are also sometimes used to elevate a tumor above nerves, periosteum, or perichondrium (ballooning) so that freezing can be extended below the tumor without harming these structures.

Complete operating-room-type aseptic technique is not a requirement, thus cryosurgery of malignant lesions can be performed in the treatment room of the physician's office, a hospital room, a nursing home, or at the patient's home. The physician can perform cryosurgery without any assistance, although a nurse or assistant can greatly facilitate the entire procedure.

Depending on the location of the lesion, the patient can be treated either lying down or in an upright position. Disabled patients or those confined to wheelchairs do not need to be transferred to the examination table. The sitting position permits downward run-off of liquid nitrogen from the area treated, and when treating trunk lesions it also allows droplets from the tip of the spray nozzle to drop harmlessly out of the way. When lesions of the inner canthus or below the eye are treated, the patient should be sitting or lying with a headrest to elevate the top of the head, so that any possible run-off would be away from the eye.

It is essential to shield vital areas from the direct spray, accumulation, or run-off of liquid nitrogen. Protective devices include styrofoam, wooden tongue blade, plastic spoons, cotton, goggles, and the Jaeger-lid retractor (see Fig. 3-10). All of these items, along with others, can be used with improvisation. The manner in which these items are used is described later in this chapter in relationship to treatment of specific areas.

The site to be treated may be cleansed with alcohol or a bactericidal solution, such as benzalkonium chloride 1/750 aqueous. It is advisable not to drape the treated site to allow full visualization of the area. This is important as droplets of liquid nitrogen can run beneath the drape, hidden from view, causing unwarranted freezing of healthy tissue.

Biopsy of a Lesion

Several types of instruments are useful to perform a cutaneous biopsy. These include the scalpel, curette, scissor, punch, and cutting current. The choice of which to use depends on the type of lesion, location, and personal preference of the operator. The tumor site should be cleansed with an antibacterial solution, and a small amount of local anesthetic, such as 1 to 2 percent lidocaine, is injected. After the specimen has been taken, it is imperative to obtain hemostasis. This is possible with simple pressure, use of hemostyptic agent such as 70 percent aluminum chloride, by electrocoagulation, or by use of an actual cautery.

While obtaining a biopsy it is also possible to reduce the tumor size, called debulking. Under local anesthesia exophytic or papular lesions are excised with a scalpel to the level of the skin (tangential excision) or even slightly below the normal skin (saucerization excision.) This tissue is submitted for pathologic examination. Ulcerated or necrotic lesions may be debulked by curetting the friable tissue to obtain biopsy specimens. Hemostatis is obtained by electrocoagulation or application of 70 percent aluminum chloride solution.

Biopsies are usually taken before treatment because the findings during gross examination of the biopsy site and the microscopic examination can influence the type and amount of cryosurgical treatment. If there is any doubt about the diagnosis, cryosurgery is postponed until the microscopic diagnosis is reported. If the clinical diagnosis is not in doubt, a specimen can be taken immediately before treatment. The histologic findings will later confirm the clinician's working diagnosis. It is possible to obtain the specimen immediately after the lesion has been treated cryosurgically. This prevents bleeding at the biopsy site, and allows even freezing of the lesion, which is particularly indicated if a punch-type biopsy is desired. Biopsies can also be taken after complete healing has occurred to determine whether any cancerous tissue is still present. Small (2 mm) punches are adequate for this purpose.

Removal of excess tissue helps define the margins of the tumor making it easier to treat cryosurgically. The thinner the lesion, the more accurately one can determine the depth dose by clinical methods. It is also simpler to place thermocouples or electrodes in thin lesions.

Spray Techinque

The spray technique is most commonly used. It consists of spraying liquid nitrogen at the lesion, under low pressure, from a distance of 1 to 2 cm through nozzles or needles (16 to 22 gauge). The spray should be applied evenly to the surface of the lesion, but not to the skin surrounding the lesion. This can be carried out in two ways: (a) as a direct open spray without a surface barrier and (b) as a restricted spray in conjunction with the use of a surface barrier such as neoprene or otoscope cones to confine the spray.

Open-Spray Technique

The open-spray technique is easily learned and produces rapid freezing of tissue. It is suitable for lesions of any size or shape including flat, exophytic, or ulcerative lesions. It is the best technique for treatment of irregularly shaped lesions, multiple skin cancers, wide lesions, tumors located at difficult sites, and curved areas such as the shoulders, ears, and nose. The amount of the cryogen delivered to the lesion can be regulated by changing the diameter of the nozzle opening and by intermittent application. This technique can be used in conjunction with curettage or partial excision. There is a minimum of destruction of healthy tissue when the open-spray technique is used as the spray can be directed to conform to the outline of the tumor. Because a surface limiting device is not used, the spray apparatus can be moved freely so that one can easily follow the outline of the tumor (Fig. 7-1)

There are some disadvantages when using the open-spray technique. The depth of freeze in relation to the lateral spread of freeze is shallower, and thick lesions may need to be debulked before treatment. Accumulation of liquid nitrogen droplets, particularly at the inner canthus or at the external auditory canal, may occur as freezing progresses, especially with certain cryosurgical units; therefore, these sites should be protected. Cryospray forms vapors, which can be a problem when working in a confined area as the operator's vision may be obscured.

Restricted-Spray Technique

The spray can be used in association with a surface barrier that confines the spray to a specific area. The liquid nitrogen is sprayed directly into the larger opening of a neoprene truncated cone while the smaller opening is held firmly against the skin (Fig. 7-2). These cones can be molded to fit the lesion, and are available in various sizes. This technique has been described in the literature as the cone-spray technique. An otoscope cone can be used in a similar manner. An advantage to the use of these surface barriers is that the lateral spread of freeze can be judged more closely. Use of these devices aid in establishing proper lateral spread of freeze dimensions, and thus more accurate estimation of the depth of freeze.

Closed Cryoprobe

The cryoprobe technique uses a hollow metal cylinder that is cooled from within by a constant flow of liquid nitrogen. It is most suitable for small- or medium-sized lesions (less than 2 cm) and those that are roughly round in shape (Fig. 7-3). It is difficult to use a cryoprobe for irregularly shaped lesions. For large lesions, multiple applications are necessary. It can be used to advantage for ulcerative lesions located on the face to avoid the possibility of gas insufflation into the subcutaneous tissue. The depth of freeze can be greater with this technique as one is able to compress the tissue during freezing. The danger of liquid nitrogen run-off or accumulation of droplets is eliminated when a cryoprobe is used. Treatment, however, is slower than with spray as the cryogen must first cool the probe before the tissue can be frozen.

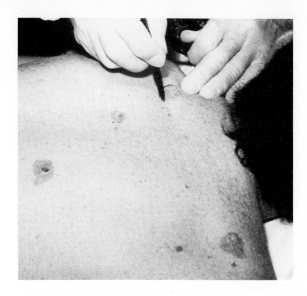

Figure 7-1. Open-spray technique. **A.** Marking margins of superficial basal cell carcinoma.

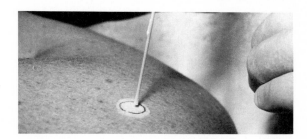

Figure 7-1B. Evenly freezing surface of lesion.

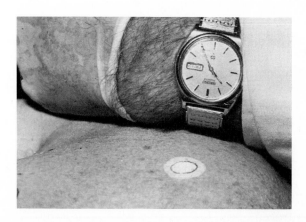

Figure 7-1C. Freezing complete. Note lateral spread of freeze. Clocking halo thaw time.

The cryoprobe is used in two manners: either in contact with the skin surface or placed intralesionally. For the surface freezing technique, where no wound is caused, a flat probe is commonly used and a rounded cryoprobe can be used for deep tumors or after curettage. Pointed cryoprobes are not commonly used in the treatment of malignancies. Cryoprobes are available in various diameters. To facilitate heat transfer during freezing, a good bond between the probe and the tissue is necessary. Wetting the skin or applying petrolatum or K-Y jelly before the application of the probe aides bonding. During freezing, the probe becomes adherent to the tissue; any movement will interfere with the heat transfer.

A less commonly used technique is the intralesional application of a cryoprobe. It is used by general surgeons and rarely by dermatologists. It is indicated for soft tumors or deep lesions; a round-ended or flat probe can be used, which produces freezing of the tissue along the sides as well as the bottom of the probe. The freezing time should be measured, but the lateral spread of freezing is not monitored. Instrumental depth dose monitoring is necessary with this technique.

Open-End Cryoprobe

In the open-end cryoprobe technique, which is not recommended by us but used by some cryosurgeons, a hollow tube is attached directly to the cryosurgical instrument and liquid nitrogen is delivered into this open-end hollow cylinder. The spray is directed so that it is continuously spraying in the center. It forms an iceball (freezing pattern) that is deeper for the same width than with the restricted spray method (in which intermittent spray is evenly applied to the surface). With this method, lateral spread of freeze measurements do not relate to depth of freeze as with the open spray, cone spray, or closed cryoprobe methods. If this method is used without thermocouple monitoring, the iceball pattern of each open-end probe applicator should be well understood by laboratory testing before application on patients.

TREATMENT OF SHALLOW LESIONS

Although cutaneous malignancies vary greatly in size, depth, and shape, most are not deeply invasive. From the cryosurgical point of view, a shallow lesion is one that does not extend more than 3 mm below the skin surface. The depth of the lesion can be ascertained through palpation, visualization, curettage, or through removal of portions of the lesion for biopsy. A suspected neoplasm should be biopsied and the specimen submitted for histologic examination. For small papular lesions a rounded scalpel (#15) blade can be used to *saucerize* the lesion while obtaining tissue for histologic examination. If the clinical diagnosis leaves doubt, the physician can proceed with

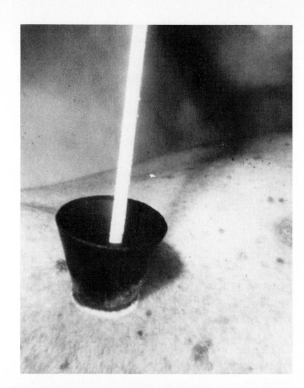

Figure 7-2. Restricted-spray technique. Neoprene cone used to limit spray to lesion surface. Note halo appearing peripheral to the cone.

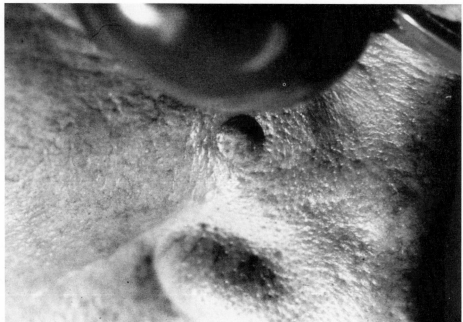

Figure 7-3. Cryoprobe technique. **A.** Lesion lateral to nose.

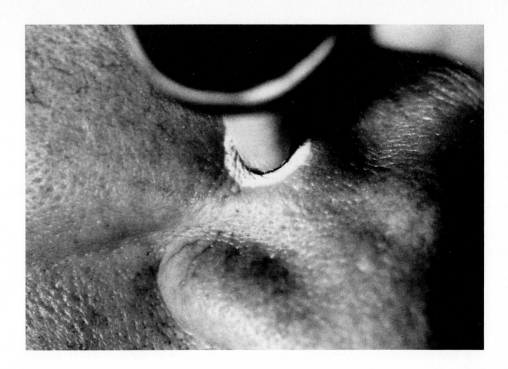

Figure 7-3B. Lesion frozen.

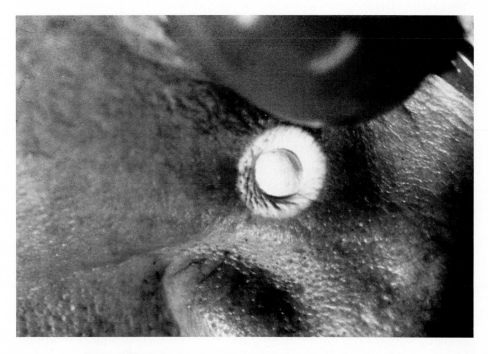

Figure 7-3C. Freezing complete. Note lateral spread of freeze.

cryosurgery immediately after taking the biopsy. Freezing is initiated and the clinical monitoring factors are observed and measured. The depth of freeze is related to the lateral spread of freeze. When the lateral spread of freeze within the appropriate freeze time has been reached, further freezing is discontinued. The use of instrument monitoring is not a requirement as it is for deeper lesions, but may be used as an added check. Generally, a double freeze–thaw cycle is carried out; however, a single freeze–thaw cycle may suffice when treating small shallow lesions.

TREATMENT OF DEEPER LESIONS

Basal and squamous cell carcinomas have the propensity to enlarge, both laterally and in depth. For cryosurgical purposes, a deeper lesion is one that extends more than 3 mm below the skin surface. It is essential to determine the depth and margins of a deeper neoplasm before treatment. Depending on the type, depth, and location of the lesion, the cryosurgeon can select the proper technique of freezing.

The treatment of deeper lesions frequently requires the use of instrument monitoring, as well as the observation and measurement of the aforementioned clinical factors. There are two different methods of instrument monitoring. The tissue temperature at the frozen site can be measured using thermocouple-tipped needles that are connected to a pyrometer. The needles are inserted at an angle from a point lateral to the tumor and the thermocouple may suffice when treating a small tumor, but in the case of wider lesions, two or more thermocouple needles are necessary to assure that adequate treatment is obtained (Fig. 7-4). For segmental treatment, a thermocouple can be reimplanted at different sites as treatment progresses. The thermocouple needle may be inserted at a predetermined depth by use of a template or a clamp. An alternate method of monitoring involves inserting the thermocouple needle vertically at the margin of the tumor. The temperature that must be attained for eradication of cancerous tissue lies between −30C to −60C, depending on the size, type, depth, and location of the lesion. Temperatures of −50C to −60C are needed for tumors that extend into the subcutaneous tissue or for those that have the potential to metastasize.

When using the thermocouple–pyrometer system the determination of adequate treatment is accomplished by a combination of the desired temperature, freezing for the proper length of time, and obtaining the halo, as an interrelationship exists between the freeze time, the lateral spread of freeze, and the depth of freeze. When this point is reached, freezing is halted and the tissue is allowed to thaw completely. A second freeze–thaw cycle is then carried out to insure a higher cure rate.

The electrical resistance method for monitoring cryosurgical treatment requires the use of an ohmmeter (Fig. 7-5). Special apparatus designed for cryosurgical use has not yet been approved by the Food and Drug Adminis-

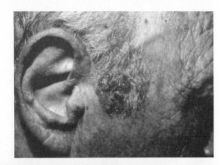

Figure 7-5. Electrical resistance technique. **A.** Basal cell carcinoma anterior to the ear.

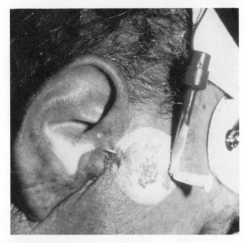

Figure 7-5B. Lesion frozen with curved needle Cradling technique of active electrode placement.

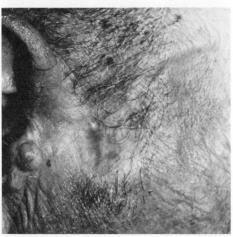

Figure 7-5C. Scar 2 months after treatment.

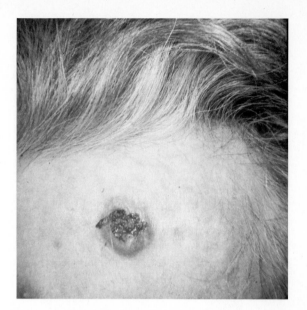

Figure 7-6. Combined technique. **A.** Basal cell carcinoma of forehead.

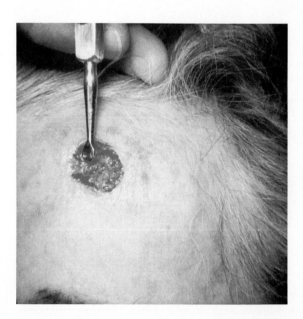

Figure 7-6B. Curettage of exophytic portion.

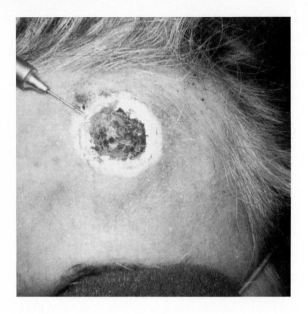

Figure 7-6C. Lesion frozen by open spray. Thermocouple needle inserted to monitor base.

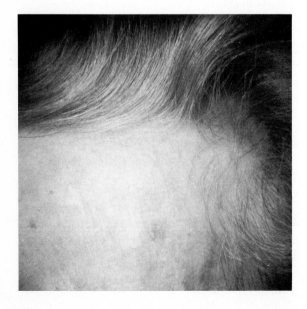

Figure 7-6D. Area completely healed.

lesion can be treated in one visit by dividing the lesion into 2 cm sections and freezing each segment consecutively as previously described. If thermocouple needles are used, they can be reimplanted under each segment as treatment progresses. Wide, irregularly shaped lesions can easily be treated in this fashion or, the surgeon can treat only a portion of the lesion, allowing it to heal, and then continue treatment on the remaining sections of the tumor at a later time. Overlapping of freezing does not hinder wound healing. By dividing the treatment of a large lesion, the acute morbidity can be reduced, although the overall healing time is longer.

PALLIATIVE TREATMENT

Cryosurgery is also useful for palliative therapy of malignant lesions. The cryosurgeon can offer patients with inoperable tumors a treatment modality that is beneficial although not curative. It may be more suitable in certain cases than extensive surgical excision or radiation therapy.

After freezing, the treated site sloughs away allowing some healing at the site. This can result in reduction of the tumor mass, avoidance of infection, amelioration of pain, and elimination of foul odors or bleeding. It facilitates nursing care and can improve the cosmetic appearance of the patient. An important consideration, in some cases, is that the patient's family is happier after palliative treatment.

It is possible to treat cutaneous metastatic lesions, although distant metastases are not affected by cryosurgical treatment. If necessary, chemotherapy can also be combined with cryosurgery.

TREATMENT OF MULTIPLE LESIONS

Cryosurgery is very useful for eradication of multiple tumors due to the simplicity of treatment, the avoidance of considerable excisional surgery, and the low cost and satisfactory cosmetic results. The lesions that most commonly develop in multiple fashion are papulonodular lesions, ulcerative tumors, superficial basal cell carcinomas, and nevoid tumors. The lesions may be scattered on the body or several may be concentrated at one anatomic area.

The cryosurgical management consists of either freezing several lesions at the same time, or freezing individual lesions at subsequent visits. The technique of treatment does not vary from that previously described. Regardless of the number of lesions treated, the depth of freezing must be adapted for each tumor according to its particular characteristics (location, size, depth, recurrence).

There may be increased morbidity if several lesions are treated at the

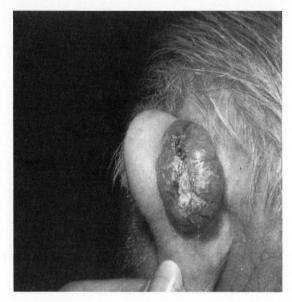

Figure 7-7. Debulking. **A.** Large exophytic lesion posterior to the ear.

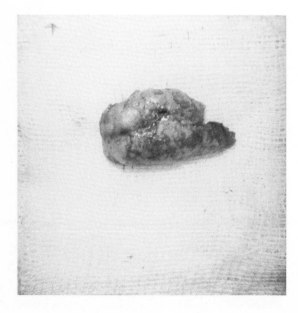

Figure 7-7B. Excised exophytic portion of the tumor.

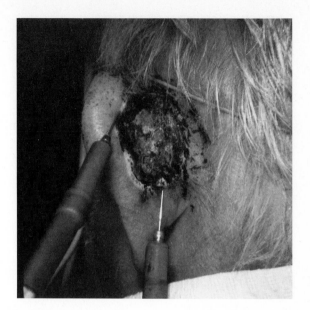

Figure 7-7C. Cryosurgical treatment started with two thermo-couple needles in place.

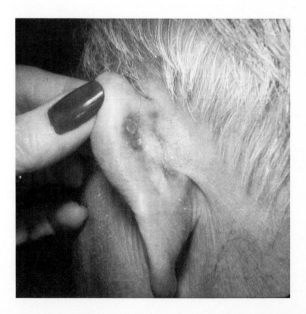

Figure 7-7D. Tumor site 6 weeks postoperative.

same time. It is not obligatory to wait until complete healing has occurred before treating additional lesions. Overlapping of freezing may occur when lesions are in close proximity to one another but this does not adversely affect wound healing. Cryosurgery can be used for the eradication of selected tumors, whereas others can be eradicated by the use of other modalities.

TREATMENT OF RECURRENT LESIONS

Several factors are involved when considering cryosurgical treatment for recurrent lesions; namely, definable borders, depth of penetration, size and location, type of tumor, and previous form of therapy. Although only selected recurrent lesions are candidates for cryosurgical management, those that present with recognizable or palpable borders can be eradicated.

A curette can aid in seeking out the margins of the tumor, or it may be necessary to obtain more than one biopsy from the margins of the lesion to determine the extent of the tumor.

Treatment must be carried out in a vigorous manner; the lateral spread of freeze should extend 5 to 10 mm beyond the margins of the tumor, the depth of freeze should be between −50C and −60C, and a double freeze–thaw cycle should be carried out. In some instances, a triple freeze–thaw cycle is beneficial. If the tumor is bound to cartilage, the thermocouple needle is inserted into the cartilaginous tissue and the iceball extended into it.

In the case of a recurrent tumor, any scar tissue that is present may be part of the recurrence and should be outlined with a marker and included in the total area to be treated. It should be emphasized that the cure rate is lower whenever treating recurrent lesions.

TREATMENT OF TUMORS AT VARIOUS ANATOMIC LOCATIONS

Facial and Neck Lesions

Facial and neck lesions account for the majority of cutaneous malignancies. Many can be eradicated with cryosurgery with good results. The techniques of treatment have been outlined and generally are applicable without modification.

Tumors on the cheeks and neck respond in a predictable fashion and the cure rate is high. The patient should be forewarned of the possible development of edema at the periorbital or mandibular areas, depending on the location of the tumor. The cosmetic results are acceptable, although hypopigmentation can be a drawback.

Tumors on the face can vary in depth and size, thus the guidelines for treatment of shallow and deep lesions should be observed.

Tumors on the chin can penetrate deeply, and therefore, the cosmetic results might not be as good in this area. Hypertrophic scarring can occur at the philtrum, and cryosurgery may not be considered as the treatment of choice in this area.

Tumors on the upper lip and near the corners of the mouth can lead to scarring and asymmetry through retraction. Lesions at the paranasal areas can extend onto the nose and may undermine tissue, therefore, these tumors should be thoroughly investigated before treatment. Malignancies that occur at the preauricular area may extend onto the tragus and cryosurgery can be used to advantage in such cases; however, ulcerative lesions can penetrate deeply in this area and cryosurgery may not be indicated.

Scalp and Forehead Lesions

Good results can be expected with properly selected cases on the scalp and forehead (Fig. 7-8).

Forehead and scalp tumors are treated with the same techniques as described earlier, but many require some modification. Because of the thickness of the scalp, malignancies may penetrate deeply and require more aggressive treatment. A double or triple freeze–thaw cycle should be carried out, and the temperature at the base of the lesion should reach −50C to −60C. For deep lesions the iceball should also be fixed to the periosteum and remain fixed for at least 1 minute. A pressure ring can be applied around the tumor during freezing to prevent oozing of blood. As a safety factor, ballooning may be used to lift the skin away from the bone.

When treating forehead lesions the eyes should be protected with proper shielding such as application of a clean plastic spoon over the globe. Also, the patient should be forewarned that a migraine-type headache may occur and persist for several hours. As mentioned earlier, periorbital edema may develop.

Penetrating lesions on the scalp and forehead should be examined thoroughly because they can invade into the periosteum. Tumors that extend to this depth may also spread laterally along the periosteum, indicating wide and deep biopsies, and generous margins during the aggressive treatment. X-rays may be indicated in the case of a deep tumor to investigate whether invasion of bone by cancerous tissue has occurred; such cases are best treated by Moh's chemosurgery.

Nose Lesions

Many tumors on the nose respond well to cryosurgery. Only those lesions that have recognizable borders are the best candidates for cryosurgical treatment (Fig. 7-9). If the lesion is ulcerated, every attempt should be made to ascertain the depth of penetration. This can be accomplished through visual examination, palpation, curettage, or finger examination through the nares. Careful examination should be made of ulcerative lesions that extend to the inner canthus, and x-rays may be indicated to determine if the tumor has penetrated into bony tissue. In the case of irregularly shaped lesions, it may

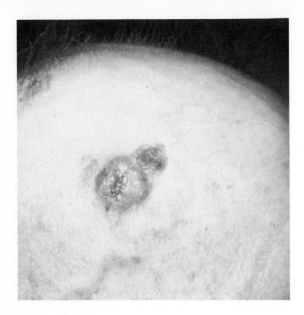

Figure 7-8A. Scalp lesion in 77-year-old man.

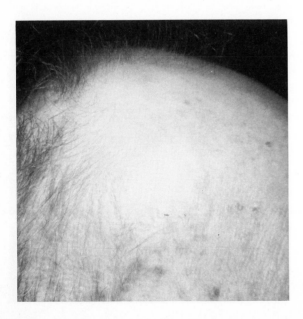

Figure 7-8B. Five-year follow-up.

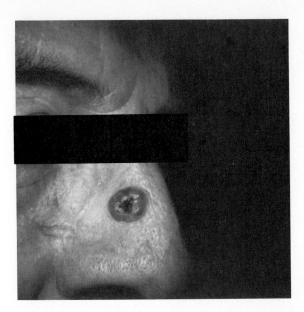

Figure 7-9A. Nodular pigmented basal cell carcinoma of the nose.

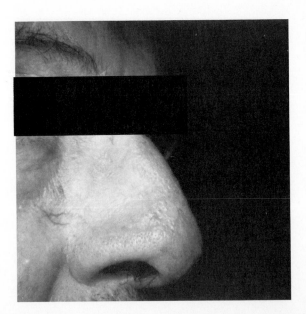

Figure 7-9B. Result 3.5 years after cryosurgery.

be necessary to take more than one biopsy to determine the extent of the lesion.

The treatment of malignancies on the nose is similar to that of facial lesions. The local anesthetic is frequently used to lift the lesion (ballooning) away from the cartilage or bone. Thermocouple needles are inserted in the usual manner, but can also be implanted through the nares. If the tumor has penetrated into cartilage, deep freezing can successfully eradicate it by extending the iceball into the cartilage.

Oftentimes, plastic or firm rubber goggles are used to protect the eyes when freezing a lesion on the nose. Soft cotton can be inserted into the nares when treating tumors at the tip of the nose and nasolabial area.

Cartilage is generally spared from damage by freezing. If invasion by cancerous tissue has already occurred, the cartilage will not be restored exactly to its normal contour after treatment. Treatment near the nares may result in cartilage defect with or without involvement by the tumor.

Lesions located at the tip of the nose are often the papular and noduloulcerative varieties. They may extend to the nostrils or wrap around the entire bulb of the nose. An open-spray technique, with or without a surface barrier, is suitable for tumors at this location. Hypopigmented depressed scars can be expected with deep lesions.

Lesions located at the nasolabial folds should be sharply demarcated if cryosurgery is undertaken. Because of the uneven contours and confluence of surgical planes at this site, treatment should be vigorous. Use of a small (1- to 2-mm) curette in the nasolabial fold area is helpful in finding deep tracts of tumor tissue.

Selected cases of tumors on the free edge or just inside the nares can be treated by cryosurgery, particularly with the spray techniques. This can sometimes preclude a large excision and reconstructive procedure that might otherwise be necessary. Slight notching or retraction, however, can occur on healing.

Eyelid Lesions

Malignancies of the eyelids account for approximately 4 percent of all cutaneous neoplasms and 45 percent of all malignant ocular tumors. The types of tumors that develop include basal cell and squamous cell carcinomas, basosquamous cell carcinoma, sebaceous carcinoma, intraepithelial epithelioma, and malignant melanoma. The most frequent tumor encountered is basal cell carcinoma, which accounts for 95 percent of the malignancies, and occurs mainly on the lower lid. The clinical types of basal cell carcinomas that are encountered on the lids are the papular, nodular, ulcerative, cystic, sclerosing, multicentric, and recurrent types.

Cryosurgery can be a treatment of choice for many eyelid tumors located at the canthi, tarsal, or orbital sections, but should not be undertaken by the novice. The spray techniques are preferred for the treatment of lid lesions. Instrument monitoring is usually indicated (Fig. 7-10).

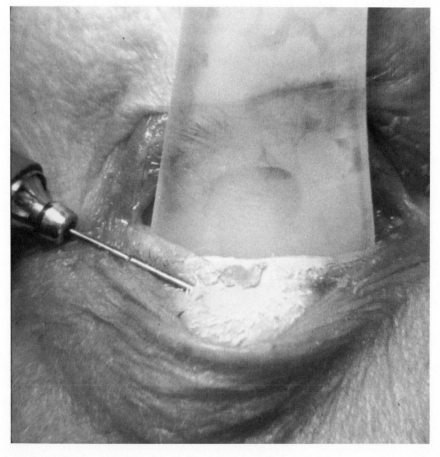

Figure 7-10. Thermocouple needle placed below eyelid lesion. Open-spray technique. Note plastic retractor used to protect globe.

For tumors on the lid margin, a spray or probe technique may be used. Treatment of small lesions can be carried into the tarsal plate usually without disturbing normal function or causing distortion of the lid. The eyeball is protected by use of a sterile Jaeger retractor placed in the conjunctional sac between the lid and the globe. Insulated chalazion clamps are useful when treating some lid lesions. A rapid acting anesthetic, such as proparacaine hydrochloride (Opthaine solution) may be instilled before the protective device is put in place. A metal shield should not be used, as it can act as a conductor. The opposite eye should also be protected from any accidental application of liquid nitrogen. When treating lesions located on the margins of the lid, a nonpurulent conjunctivitis usually develops. This condition can be relieved with the use of an antibiotic ophthalmic solution.

Cryosurgery of lesions near the punctum and lacrimal duct should be carefully monitored. The lacrimal duct usually recovers from mild freezing but can be permanently damaged by very low temperatures. Lesions located at the inner canthus should be carefully examined to determine localization. Malignancies may invade deeply at this location and extend behind the orbit. Recurrence of a tumor in this area is a very serious matter, and can result in loss of vision or death. If the borders of the tumor are indistinct, such tumors should not be treated with cryosurgery but referred for other management.

Ear Lesions

Cutaneous malignancies may arise on any portion of the ear. They can be of any size, and can remain within the skin or penetrate into the underlying cartilage. One should attempt to determine whether the tumor is fixed to the cartilage by palpation or by the taking of a 2-mm punch biopsy. If the tumor rises above the cartilage after the use of local anesthetic, then it is not fixed to the cartilage. This is an important step as the amount of treatment and the outcome are determined, in part, by the depth and penetration of the tumor.

The cryosurgical management of tumors on the ear is basically the same as previously described, but might necessitate modifications. Consideration has to be given to the curvature of the ear, the presence of cartilage, the lack of subcutaneous tissue, and the auditory canal. Furthermore, a tumor may involve both the anterior and posterior aspects of the ear.

The spray techniques are best, except for small, round lesions, which can be treated with the cryoprobe. The spray should conform to the shape of the lesion and the curvature of the ear (Figs. 7-11 and 7-12). To minimize the chance of a recurrence, inadequate freezing is to be avoided. Monitoring the temperature at the margins of a tumor may sometimes be indicated, rather than monitoring the depth. If the tumor is not fixed to cartilage, the lesion is lifted away from the cartilage with a local anesthetic (ballooning), and the thermocouple needle is inserted between the tumor and the cartilage. If the tumor does invade the cartilage, then the thermocouple needle is placed on

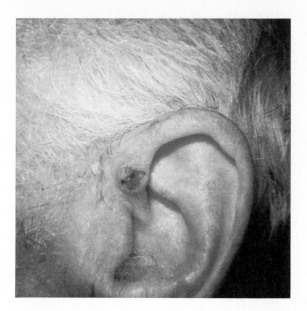

Figure 7-11A. Basal cell carcinoma of crus helicus.

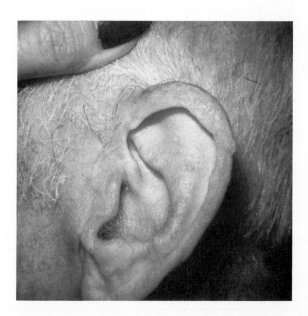

Figure 7-11B. Result 14 months postoperative. Note slight notching.

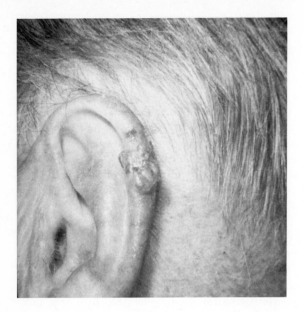

Figure 7-12A. Nodular basal cell carcinoma of helix.

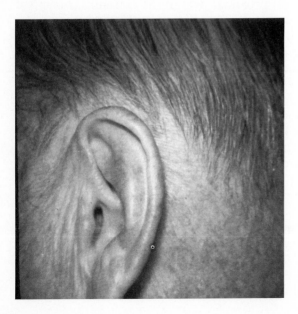

Figure 7-12B. Result 1 year post-operative.

the other side of the cartilage, and the freeze allowed to extend through the cartilage. When confronted with more than one tumor on an ear, it is wise to treat one lesion and allow it to heal for 2 to 3 weeks before treating the next to avoid severe or prolonged edema.

Most areas on the ear respond well. The results of treatment at the helix are excellent, but one should be cautioned about possible cartilage loss, which occasionally occurs. Cryosurgery produces very good results when used at the lobe and the normal architecture is retained. Good results can be expected at the posterior crease in selected cases. One should treat with caution linear-type lesions that proceed up or down the crease. It is essential to protect the ear canal from inadvertent spraying of liquid nitrogen or accumulation of liquid nitrogen droplets. A cotton–wool pledget is placed in the ear canal before cryosurgery.

One must be cautious in dealing with ulcerative or nodular tumors at the preauricular area, because lesions here have the potential to invade deeply. A liberal amount of anesthetic should be injected before treatment of a lesion in this area to lift the skin. If a tumor extends into the auditory canal, treatment should be undertaken only by an expert and in conjunction with an otolaryngologist who can biopsy the site after healing to determine the success of treatment. One should also be careful of certain lesions that seem to find a deeper facial plane and can run inferiorly or superiorly near the margins of the cartilage of the ear. These should be very cautiously, if at all, treated by cryosurgical means.

Trunk and Extremity Lesions

Tumors located on the trunk and proximal part of the extremities respond well to crysurgery, but with a longer healing time (6 to 12 weeks).

Treatment is performed in the usual manner, but in the case of large lesions the guidelines for segmental treatment can be applied. With the absence of vital tissues, excluding the nipples and genitalia, a lesion can be frozen with the inclusion of a wide margin of normal-appearing surrounding skin to insure a higher cure rate. Depending on the size and shape of the lesion, either the spray technique or cryoprobe technique can be employed. The open spray is best for large or irregularly shaped lesions. In such cases, it is necessary to implant more than one thermocouple needle to monitor the depth of freezing. Oftentimes a bullous reaction develops that may be of some discomfort to the patient.

An advantage of cryosurgery is that it can be used to eradicate multiple lesions, such as superficial basal cell carcinomas or nevoid tumors, at one visit. Cryosurgery is particularly useful for lesions that curve around the shoulders and extremities. In general, the upper extremities do well both as to cure rates and cosmetic results. Some amount of caution is necessary on the dorsum of the hand, and extreme caution is advised where nerves lie superficially, as around the ulnar fossa and the lateral sides of the fingers.

Injection of large amounts of local anesthetic to balloon the skin away from these structures is indicated. Prolonged healing usually accompanies cryosurgery of malignant lesions on the lower portions of the legs, and the incidence of secondary infection is higher. These drawbacks also apply to most alternate procedures performed in this area.

LENTIGO MALIGNA

Lentigo maligna is considered a precancerous type of lesion by most dermatologists but as an in situ malignant melanoma by some. It is an intraepidermal process with atypical melanocytes extending not only horizontally, but also vertically to the hair follicles and adnexal tissue. The diagnosis should be confirmed histologically.

Cryosurgery is indicated if the lesion is in a location or of a size so that simple excision and closure is not advisable, or excision is contraindicated for some other reason. Only completely flat lesions are to be treated (Fig. 7-13). The objective is to eliminate all the melanocytes. Lesions with any nodular element should be considered potential melanoma (lentigo maligna melanoma) and should be excised for complete microscopic examination. Treatment of lentigo maligna consists of deep freezing and the use of instrumentation monitoring. The cryoprobe or open-spray techniques are suitable. The entire lesion and at least a 10-mm peripheral border of healthy skin must be frozen so that all the melanocytes in the site, including those in the hair follicles, receive a lethal dose. A temperature of approximately −30C at a level of 3 mm must be attained. The monitoring can be done effectively by thermocouple needles or electrodes to the level of the hair bulbs. A double freeze–thaw cycle is preferred by most cryosurgeons. A *biological marker* for evaluating adequate treatment is healing with a nonpigmented scar. Recurrence of even normal pigmentation in the area of the lentigo maligna signifies that treatment is inadequate to destroy all the melanocytes. A small rim of repigmentation may occur, however, from migration of melanocytes from healthy tissue surrounding the lesion.

GENERAL RESULTS

Cryosurgical treatment of malignant lesions produces a rapid and predictable response. The healing times vary according to size, depth, and location of the lesion. The appearance of a treated site immediately after complete healing shows a temporary redness. On the whole, facial lesions including ear, nose, eyelid, and neck, heal completely in approximately 4 to 6 weeks, whereas trunk lesions require more time. Lower extremity lesions may take even longer.

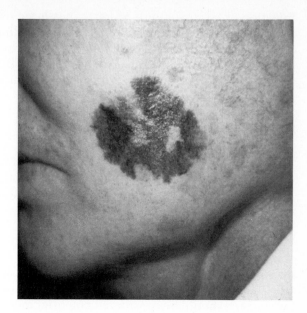

Figure 7-13A. Lentigo maligna of the cheek.

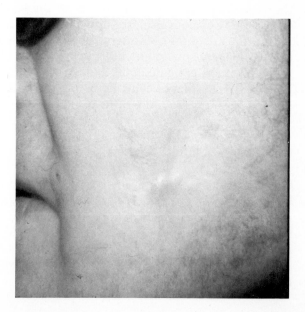

Figure 7-13B. Site at 5 months.

POSTOPERATIVE COURSE AND AFTERCARE

Shortly after treatment, urtication and edema begins. It can range from mild to severe, the swelling depends to a great extent on the location of the tumor. Within 24 hours an exudative reaction ensues. This may vary in intensity and depends on the depth of freeze, the size of tumor, and the host response. It generally lasts for approximately 3 to 10 days for lesions on the face and the head, and longer for lesions located on the trunk or the extremities. This reaction may be of some discomfort to the patient, but is generally well tolerated. Toward the latter part of the exudative period the site begins to dry and sloughing occurs. This, in turn, is followed by the development of a crust that eventually loosens and falls away spontaneously.

The aftercare for treated malignant lesions corresponds to the stages of reaction to deep freezing as mentioned previously. Dry gauze dressings are applied during the exudative stage. Normal cleansing of the site with soap and water, hydrogen peroxide, or benzalconium chloride aqueous solution 1:750 is recommended. If edema is present, cold water compresses are helpful. When a crust forms the patient is advised to apply alcohol, or the above-mentioned solutions once or twice daily with a cotton ball until complete healing occurs. During this stage a dressing is optional.

CURE RATE

In treating skin cancer cure rate is the primary criterion for selecting the modality to be used, although end functional and cosmetic results are important, secondary factors are cost and time. Cryosurgery has been used for over 20 years, therefore, adequate long-term statistics are available based on treatment of many thousands of lesions. During this period Zacarian has reported on over 4000 lesions and Graham on over 2000 lesions. The authors of this book, Torre, Lubrits, and Kuflik have treated more than 5000 lesions.

Zacarian's overall cure rate of 97.3 percent consists of 15 percent of lesions followed under 3 years, 25 percent 3 to 5 years, 60 percent 5 years or longer. His recurrence rate is not even over the 5-year period, 43.3 percent of recurrences were within the first year, 24.3 percent in the second year, 19 percent in the third year, and only 3.4 percent after third year. To convert his figures into 5-year follow-up statistics, cure rate on 40 percent of his cases would have to be factored down to represent expected recurrences. This would bring his cure rate figures to slightly below 97 percent for 5 years in comparison with other methods. Graham reports an overall cure rate of 95.57 percent. This would also have to be factored down to express 5-year cure rates. Torre, Lubritz, and Kuflik, without detailed analysis, have 5-year cure rates that also fit into the 95 to 97 percent range, therefore, it reasonable to give this 95 to 97 percent figure as a 5-year cure target. This compares favorably to 5-year cure rates by all methods except Moh's chemosurgery as

TABLE 7-1. TECHNIQUES OF TREATMENT

Mark margins of the tumor. Measure the diameter and record.

Inject local analgesia. Balloon if indicated.

Biopsy if not previously done. Obtain hemostasis.

A. Open Spray Technique
1. Select nozzle suitable for lesion (for deep lesion insert thermocouple and/or resistance electrode).
2. Spray tumor evenly on surface until freezing spreads peripherally into healthy tissue for a radius of 5-mm (LSF 5-mm).
3. Record freeze time (should be 60–90 sec).
   For shallow lesions record halo thaw time (should be over 60 sec). For deep lesions continue to freeze until pyrometer reads −50C and/or ohmmeter reads 5 megaohms.

B. Restricted Spray Technique (cone-spray)
1. Select truncated neoprene cone with small end opening slightly larger than the lesion diameter. (For deep lesions insert thermocouple needle and/or resistance electrode.)
2. Spray evenly onto surface enclosed by cone until frozen rim appears 1.5–2 mm beyond cone. As cone is 3–3.5 mm thick, this represents a lateral spread of freeze of 5 mm. If this cone, such as an otoscope cone, is used rim should be 4–4.5 mm in radius beyond the cone.
3. For thin lesions record freeze time and allow to thaw, recording halo thaw time. For thick lesions continue freezing until pyrometer reads −50C and/or ohmmeter reads 5 megaohms.

C. Cryoprobe Technique
1. Select flat cryoprobe with base slightly larger than the diameter of the tumor, apply K-Y jelly to the tumor surface. (For deep lesions insert thermocouple needle and/or resistance electrodes.)
2. Prechill probe and apply firmly to surface.
3. For shallow lesions allow halo of freezing to extend 5 mm beyond probe. For deep lesions continue freezing until LSF is 5 mm and temperature is −50C and/or resistance 5 megaohms.
4. Allow to thaw.
5. Repeat entire freeze–thaw cycle for deep lesions and shallow lesions if desired.

reported in Crissey's compilation of 13 reports on treatment by various methods of 14,114 carcinomas of the skin. Moh's chemosurgery yielded 99.1 percent cure rate, surgical excision 95.5 percent, radiation therapy 94.7 percent, and curettage and electrodesiccate 92.6 percent.

Graham's excellent computerized analyses give us insight into individual factors influencing cure rate, such as tumor size, location and histologic type, and whether the lesion was primary or recurrent. Recurrent lesions have a higher recurrence rate than primary tumors. Very little difference was seen between basal cell and squamous cell carcinomas, but morphea-type basal cell carcinomas give a lower cure rate than nodular basal cell carcinomas. When size of tumors were considered, the smaller (0.5 cm and under) and larger (over 2.5 cm) tumors had the best cure rates, the 0.6- to 1.2-cm group had an intermediate cure rate and the 1.3- to 2.4-cm size group the lowest cure rate. The fact that the larger group contained many superficial basal cell carcinomas, and that more aggressive treatment was given to large lesions may help account for these results.

Cure rate also varies with locations. Lesions on the ear, eyelid, nose, and scalp generally give lower cure rates. Graham's statistics, however, give good results for the ear and the scalp. Her results, using different methods of cryosurgical treatment including single and double freeze and curettage preceding cryosurgery, show only a small difference in cure rate. Her statistics definitely show, however, that her more recently treated cases have improved cure rates over her early cases. She attributes this factor to better case selection, standardization of methods, and improved depth dose measurement devices and techniques.

A summary of cryosurgical techniques is contain in Table 7-1.

SELECTED READING

Fraunfelder FT, Zacarian SA, Limmer BL, et al: Cryosurgery for malignancies of the eyelid. Am Acad Ophthalmol 87:461, 1980

Graham GF, Clark LC: Statistical update in cryosurgery for cancers of the skin. In Zacarian SA (ed): Cryosurgery for Skin Cancer and Cutaneous Disorders. St. Louis, C.V. Mosby, 1985, p 298

Kuflik EG: Cryosurgery for basal-cell carcinomas on the wings of the nose and in the nasolabial folds. J Dermatol Surg Oncol 7:23, 1981

Kuflik EG: Cryosurgery for treatment of large basal-cell carcinomas on the trunk. J Dermatol Surg Oncol 9:226, 1983

Kuflik EG: Cryosurgery for palliation. J Dermatol Surg Oncol 11:9, 1985

Kuflik EG: Cryosurgery for tumors of the ear. J Dermatol Surg Oncol 11:12, 1985

Kuflik EG: Cryosurgery for carcinoma of the eyelid: A 12-year experience. J Dermatol Surg Oncol 11:243, 1985

Lubritz RR: Cryosurgery management of multiple skin carcinomas. J Dermatol Surg Oncol 3:414, 1977

Spiller WF, Spiller RF: Treatment of basal cell carcinomas by a combination of curettage and cryosurgery. J Dermatol Surg Oncol 3:443, 1977

Torre D: Cryosurgery. In Andrade R, Gumport SL, Popkin GL, Reese TD, (eds): Cancer of the Skin. Philadelphia, W. B. Saunders, 1976.

Torre D: Cryosurgical treatment of epitheliomas using the cone-spray technique. J Dermatol Surg Oncol 3:432, 1977

Torre D: Cryosurgery of basal cell carcinoma. J Am Acad Dermatol 15:917, 1986

Zacarian SA: Cryosurgical treatment of lentigo maligna. Arch Dermatol 118:89, 1982

Zacarian SA: Cryosurgery of cutaneous carcinomas: An 18-year study of 3,022 patients with 4,228 carcinomas. J Am Acad Dermatol 9(6):947, 1983

Zacarian SA: Cryosurgery for cancer of the skin. In Zacarian SA (ed): Cryosurgery for Skin Cancer and Cutaneous Disorders. St. Louis, C.V. Mosby, 1985, p 96

INDEX

Italic letters following page numbers refer to tables (*t*) and figures (*f*).

Rate, freezing and thawing, 13
Reactions to cryosurgery, 53–56, 60
Recovery. *See* Postoperative course
Repigmentation, 17
Restricted-spray technique, 91, 94*f.*
    See also Cone spray technique;
    Confined spray technique;
    Neoprene cones; Otoscope
    cones; Spray technique;
    Truncated cones
Retraction, 109
Rhinophyma, 68
Roentgen-ray therapy, 87

Salivation, 72
Saucerization, 73, 74*f*, 90, 93, 98
Scalp lesions, 106, 107*f*, 118
Scarring, 59*f*, 60. *See also* Atrophy;
    Depression; Notching;
    Retraction
  acne, 67–68
  fluorocarbon sprays and, 29
  hypertrophic, 56, 58*f*, 106
Sebaceous
  carcinoma, 109
  hyperplasia, 38, 83
Seborrheic keratoses, 77, 78*f*
Segmental treatment, 98, 102, 114
Slush, carbon dioxide, 1
Spray. *See also* Cryospray; Neoprene
    cones; Otoscope cones;
    Truncated cones
  technique
    cone spray technique, 17
    confined spray technique, 64
    depth of freezing and lateral
      spread of freeze, 91
    ear lesions and, 111
    history of, 1, 4
    malignancies and, 90–91
    open-spray, 62, 64, 73, 90–91, 92*f*,
      98, 101*f*, 102, 109, 114
    patterns, 63*f*, 77
    restricted-spray, 91, 94*f*
  tips, 35, 37*f*, 38
    slit-tip accessory, 66, 67
    treating acne with, 66

Spray (*cont.*)
  unit
    CE-8 unit, 6*f*
    Lubritz-Johns "Foster Froster," 7*f*
    Torre "do-it-yourself" hand-held
      apparatus, 7*f*
    Torre prototype, 5*f*
    Zacarian C-21, 6*f*
Squamous cell carcinoma. *See*
    Carcinomas
Steatocystoma multiplex, 83
Steroids, 52, 56, 67, 68, 73, 76
Swab technique, 1, 2*f*, 62
Swimming pool granuloma, 85
Syncope, 52

Table-top units, 31, 35, 36*f*
Target
  area, 17, 44
  dose, 44–45
  temperature, 43–44
Techniques of treatment, 118*t*
Telangiectasis, 68
Temperature, 13–16
  measurement of, 45, 48
  target, 43–44
Thaw time, 62, 64. *See also* Halo thaw
    time; Total thaw time
Thermocouple. *See also* Depth dose
    measurement; Depth
    thermocouple; Pyrometer-
    thermocouple measurement
    systems
  pyrometer measurement systems,
    38, 45
  tipped needles, 101*f*
    cartilage and, 105
    ear lesions and, 104*f*, 111
    eyelid and, 83, 110
    gauge of, 45
    lentigo maligna and, 115
    nose lesions and, 109
    placement of, 4, 47*f*
    template for predetermined depth,
      45, 96
Tissue defects, 56, 60
Torre, D., 4, 48, 117
  cryoprobe spray unit, 5*f*